High-Yield™ Biostatistics

High-Yield™ Biostatistics

Anthony N. Glaser, M.D., Ph.D.

Clinical Assistant Professor,
Medical University of South Carolina
Private Practice of Family Medicine
Charleston, South Carolina

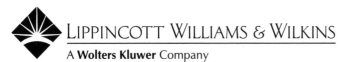

LIPPINCOTT WILLIAMS & WILKINS
A **Wolters Kluwer** Company

Philadelphia · Baltimore · New York · London
Buenos Aires · Hong Kong · Sydney · Tokyo

Editor: Elizabeth A. Nieginski
Editorial Director: Julie P. Scardiglia
Managing Editor: Marette D. Smith
Marketing Manager: Kelley Ray

351 West Camden Street
Baltimore, Maryland 21201-2436 USA

530 Walnut Street
Philadelphia, Pennsylvania 19106 USA

Printed in the United States of America

ISBN 0-781-72242-X

We'd like to hear from you! If you have comments or suggestions regarding this Lippincott Williams & Wilkins title, please contact us at the appropriate customer service number listed below, or send correspondence to **book_comments@lww.com.** If possible, please remember to include your mailing address, phone number, and a reference to the book title and author in your message. To purchase additional copies of this book call our customer service department at **(800)638-3030** or fax orders to **(301) 824-7390.** International customers should call **(301) 714-2324.**

02
3 4 5 6 7 8 9 10

To my wife, Marlene

Contents

Preface

Biostatistics is a course that most people dislike and try to scrape by on—often because it is taught by a statistician who assumes that everyone is adept at mathematics and can cope with blackboards full of formulae and equations. However, today's medical students will not, for the most part, become producers of research (and those who do will undoubtedly seek the advice of professional statisticians when designing their studies). On the other hand, all will become consumers of research and will need to understand the inferential statistical principles behind the reports that they read. Consequently, while this book does not pretend to be an in-depth statistics textbook (which few medical students have the need, the time, or the desire for), it aims to be more than a set of notes to be memorized for the purpose of examinations.

High-Yield Biostatistics explains concepts, provides examples, and also contains review exercises for the more difficult material in the first three chapters. Unlike other biostatistics books, it covers the complete range of biostatistics material that can be expected to appear on the USMLE Step 1, without going beyond that range.

The term "high yield" has become something of a buzzword among students. Its use here reflects that the core of information presented in *High-Yield Biostatistics* will be tested on the "Boards." The book contains little extraneous information, although the material does tread beyond the irreducible minimum in some instances.

For the more inquisitive reader, a small amount of additional material is presented in notes at the end of some chapters, but this information is neither necessary for a general understanding of the material nor to answer USMLE questions.

If you have any suggestions for changes or improvements to this book, or if you find a biostatistics question on Step 1 that this book does not equip you to answer, please drop me a line.

Anthony N. Glaser
tonyglaser@mindspring.com

1

Descriptive Statistics

Statistical methods fall into two broad areas: **descriptive statistics** and **inferential statistics.**

- **Descriptive statistics** merely describe, organize, or summarize data; they refer only to the actual data available. Examples include the mean blood pressure of a group of patients and the success rate of a surgical procedure.

- **Inferential statistics** involve making inferences that go beyond the actual data. They usually involve inductive reasoning (i.e., generalizing to a population after having observed only a sample). Examples include the mean blood pressure of all Americans and the expected success rate of a surgical procedure in patients who have not yet undergone the operation.

POPULATIONS, SAMPLES, AND ELEMENTS

A **population** is the universe about which an investigator wishes to draw conclusions; it need not consist of people, but may be a population of measurements. Strictly speaking, if an investigator wants to draw conclusions about the blood pressure of Americans, the population consists of the blood pressure measurements, not the Americans themselves.

A **sample** is a subset of the population—the part that is actually being observed or studied. Because researchers rarely can study whole populations, inferential statistics are almost always needed to draw conclusions about a population when only a sample has actually been studied.

A single observation—such as one person's blood pressure—is an **element,** denoted by X. The number of elements in a population is denoted by N, and the number of elements in a sample by n. A population therefore consists of all the elements from X_1 to X_N, and a sample consists of n of these N elements.

Most samples used in biomedical research are **probability samples**— samples in which the researcher can specify the probability of any one element in the population being included. For example, if someone is picking a sample of 4 playing cards at random from a pack of 52 cards, the probability that any 1 card will be included is 4/52. Probability samples permit the use of inferential statistics, whereas nonprobability samples allow only descriptive statistics to be used. There are four basic kinds of probability samples: **simple random samples, stratified random samples, cluster samples,** and **systematic samples.**

Simple random samples

The simple random sample is the simplest kind of probability sample. It is drawn in such a way that every element in the population has an equal probability of being included, such as in the playing card example above. A random sample is defined by the *method of drawing the sample*, not by the outcome. If four hearts were picked out of the pack of cards, this does not in itself mean that the sample is not random.

A sample is **representative** if it closely resembles the population from which it is drawn. All types of random samples tend to be representative, but they cannot guarantee representativeness. Nonrepresentative samples can cause serious problems. (Four hearts are clearly not representative of all the cards in a pack.)

A classic example of a nonrepresentative sample was an opinion poll taken before the 1936 U.S. Presidential Election. On the basis of a sample of more than 2 million people, it was predicted that Alfred Landon would achieve a landslide victory over Franklin Delano Roosevelt, but the result was the opposite. The problem? The sample was drawn from records of telephone and automobile ownership—people who owned such items in that Depression year were not at all representative of the electorate as a whole.

A sample or a result demonstrates **bias** if it consistently errs in a particular direction. For example, in drawing a sample of 10 from a population consisting of 500 white people and 500 black people, a sampling method that consistently produces more than 5 white people would be biased. Biased samples are therefore unrepresentative, and true randomization is proof against bias.

Stratified random samples

In a stratified random sample, the population is first divided into relatively internally homogeneous groups, or strata, from which random samples are then drawn. This stratification results in greater representativeness. For example, instead of drawing one sample of 10 people from a total population consisting of 500 white and 500 black people, one random sample of 5 could be taken from each ethnic group (or stratum) separately, thus guaranteeing the racial representativeness of the resulting overall sample of 10.

Cluster samples

Cluster samples may be used when it is too expensive or laborious to draw a simple random or stratified random sample. For example, in a survey of 100 medical students in the United States, an investigator might start by selecting a random set of groups or "clusters"—such as a random set of 10 U.S. medical schools—and then interviewing all the students in those 10 schools. This method is much more economical and practical than trying to take a random sample of 100 directly from the population of all U.S. medical students.

Systematic samples

These involve selecting elements in a systematic way—such as every fifth patient admitted to a hospital or every third baby born in a given area. This type of sampling usually provides the equivalent of a simple random sample without actually using randomization.

Sampling problems are common in clinical research.

For example, if a researcher advertises in a newspaper to recruit people suffering from a particular problem—whether it is acne, diabetes, or depression—the people who respond form a **self-selected** sample, which is probably not representative of the population of all people with this problem.

Similarly, if a dermatologist reports on the results of a new treatment for acne which he has been using with his patients, the sample may not be representative of all people with acne, as it is likely that only people with more severe acne (or with good insurance coverage!) seek treatment from a dermatologist. In any case, his practice is probably limited to people in a particular geographic, climatic, and possibly ethnic area. In this case, although his study may be valid as far as his or her patients are concerned (this is called **internal validity**), it may not be valid to generalize his findings to people with acne in general (so the study may lack **external** validity).

PROBABILITY

The **probability** of an event is denoted by **p.** Probabilities are usually expressed as decimal fractions, not as percentages, and must lie between zero (zero probability) and one (absolute certainty). The probability of an event cannot be negative. The probability of an event can also be expressed as a ratio of the number of likely outcomes to the number of possible outcomes.

> For example, if a fair coin was tossed an infinite number of times, heads would appear on 50% of the tosses; therefore, the probability of heads, or p (heads), is .50. If a random sample of 10 people was drawn an infinite number of times from a population of 100 people, each person would be included in the sample 10% of the time; therefore, p (being included in any one sample) is .10.

The probability of an event *not* occurring is equal to one minus the probability that it will occur; this is denoted by **q.** In the above example, the probability of any one person *not* being included in any one sample, (q), is therefore $(1 - p) = (1 - .10) = .90$.

> The USMLE requires familiarity with the three main methods of calculating probabilities: the addition rule, the multiplication rule, and the binomial distribution.

Addition rule

The **addition rule** of probability states that the probability of any *one* of several particular events occurring is equal to the sum of their individual probabilities, *provided* the events are mutually exclusive (i.e., they cannot *both* happen).

Because the probability of picking a heart card from a deck of cards is 0.25, and the probability of picking a diamond card is also 0.25, this rule states that the probability of picking a card that is either a heart or a diamond is $0.25 + 0.25 = 0.50$. Because no card can be both a heart and a diamond, these events meet the requirement of mutual exclusiveness.

Multiplication rule

The **multiplication rule** of probability states that the probability of two or more statistically independent events *all* occurring is equal to the product of their individual probabilities.

If the lifetime probability of a person developing cancer is 0.25, and the lifetime probability of developing schizophrenia is 0.01, the lifetime probability that a person might have *both* cancer *and* schizophrenia is $0.25 \times 0.01 = .0025$, *provided* that the two illnesses are independent—in other words, that having one illness neither increases nor decreases the risk of having the other.

Binomial distribution

The probability that a *specific combination of mutually exclusive independent events* will occur can be determined by the use of the **binomial distribution.** A binomial distribution is one in which there are only two possibilities, such as yes/no, male/female, and healthy/sick. If an experiment has exactly two possible outcomes (one of which is generally termed "success"), the binomial distribution gives the probability of obtaining an exact number of successes in a series of independent trials.

A typical medical use of the binomial distribution is in genetic counseling. Inheritance of a disorder such as Tay-Sachs disease follows a binomial distribution: there are two possible events (inheriting the disease or not inheriting it) that are mutually exclusive (one person cannot both have and not have the disease), and the possibilities are independent (if one child in a family inherits the disorder, this does not affect the chance of another child inheriting it).

A physician could therefore use the binomial distribution to inform a couple who are carriers of the disease how probable it is that some specific combination of events might occur—such as the probability that if they are to have two children, *neither* will inherit the disease. The formula for the binomial distribution does not need to be learned or used for the purposes of the USMLE.

TYPES OF DATA

The choice of an appropriate statistical technique depends on the type of data in question. Data will always form one of four **scales of measurement:** nominal, ordinal, interval, or ratio. The mnemonic "NOIR" can be used to remember these scales in order. Data may also be characterized as discrete or continuous.

Nominal   Nominal scale data are divided into qualitative categories or groups, such as male/female, black/white, urban/suburban/rural, and red/green. There is no implication of order or ratio. Nominal data that fall into only two groups are called dichotomous data.

Ordinal   Ordinal scale data can be placed in a meaningful order (e.g., students may be ranked 1st/2nd/3rd in their class). However, there is no information about the size of the interval—no conclusion can be drawn about whether the difference between the first and second students is the same as the difference between the second and third.

Interval   Interval scale data are like ordinal data in that they can be placed in a meaningful order. In addition, they have meaningful intervals between items, which are usually measured quantities. For example, on the Celsius scale the difference between 100° and 90° is the same as the difference between 50° and 40°. However, because interval scales do not have an absolute zero, ratios of scores are not meaningful: 100°C is not twice as hot as 50°C, because 0°C does not indicate a complete absence of heat.

Ratio   A ratio scale has the same properties as an interval scale; however, because it has an absolute zero, meaningful ratios do exist. Most biomedical variables form a ratio scale: weight in grams or pounds, time in seconds or days, blood pressure in millimeters of mercury, and pulse rate in beats per minute are all ratio scale data. The only ratio scale of temperature is the Kelvin scale, in which zero degrees indicates an absolute absence of heat, just as a zero pulse rate indicates an absolute lack of heartbeat. Therefore, it is correct to say that a pulse rate of 120 beats/min is twice as fast as a pulse rate of 60 beats/min, or that 300°K is twice as hot as 150°K.

Discrete   Discrete variables can take only certain values and none in between. For example, the number of patients in a hospital census may be 178 or 179, but it cannot be in between these two; the number of syringes used in a clinic on any given day may increase or decrease only by units of one.

Continuous   Continuous variables may take any value (typically between certain limits). Most biomedical variables are continuous (e.g., a patient's weight, height, age, and blood pressure). However, the process of measuring or reporting continuous variables will reduce them to a discrete variable; blood pressure may be reported to the nearest whole millimeter of mercury, weight to the nearest pound, and age to the nearest year.

FREQUENCY DISTRIBUTIONS

A set of unorganized data is difficult to digest and understand. Consider a study of the serum cholesterol levels of a sample of 200 men: a list of the 200 levels would be of little value in itself. A simple first way of organizing the data is to list all the possible values between the highest and the lowest in order, recording the frequency (f) with which each score occurs. This forms a **frequency distribution.** If the highest serum cholesterol level were 260 mg/dl, and the lowest were 161 mg/dl, the frequency distribution might be as shown in Table 1–1

Grouped frequency distributions

Table 1–1 is an unwieldy presentation of data. These data can be made more manageable by creating a **grouped frequency distribution,** shown in Table 1–2. Individual scores are grouped (between 7 and 20 groups are usually appropriate). Each group of scores encompasses an **equal class interval.** In this example there are 10 groups with a class interval of 10 (161 to 170, 171 to 180, and so on).

Relative frequency distributions

As Table 1–2 shows, a grouped frequency distribution can be transformed into a **relative frequency distribution,** which shows the *percentage* of all the elements that fall within each class interval. The relative frequency of elements in any given class interval is found by dividing f, the frequency (or number of elements) in that class interval, by n (the sample size, which in this case is 200). By multiplying the result by 100, it is converted into a percentage. Thus, this distribution shows, for example, that 19% of this sample had serum cholesterol levels between 211 and 220 mg/dl.

Cumulative frequency distributions

Table 1–2 also shows a **cumulative frequency distribution.** This is also expressed as a percentage; it shows the percentage of elements lying *within and below* each class interval. Although a group may be called the 211–220 group, this group actually includes the range of scores that lie from 210.5 up to and including 220.5—so these figures are the **exact upper** and **lower limits** of the group.

The relative frequency column shows that 2% of the distribution lies in the 161–170 group and 2.5% lies in the 171–180 group; therefore, a total of 4.5% of the distribution lies at or below a score of 180.5, as shown by the cumulative frequency column in Table 1–2. A further 6% of the distribution lies in the 181–190 group; therefore, a total of (2 + 2.5 + 6) = 10.5% lies at or below a score of 190.5. A man with a serum cholesterol level of 190 mg/dl can be told that roughly 10% of this sample had lower levels than his, and approximately 90% had scores above his. The cumulative frequency of the highest group (251–260) must be 100, showing that 100% of the distribution lies at or below a score of 260.5.

Table 1-1

Score	f	Score	f	Score	f	Score	f	Score	f
260	1	240	2	220	4	200	3	180	0
259	0	239	1	219	2	199	0	179	2
258	1	238	2	218	1	198	1	178	1
257	0	237	0	217	3	197	3	177	0
256	0	236	3	216	4	196	2	176	0
255	0	235	1	215	5	195	0	175	0
254	1	234	2	214	3	194	3	174	1
253	0	233	2	213	4	193	1	173	0
252	1	232	4	212	6	192	0	172	0
251	1	231	2	211	5	191	2	171	1
250	0	230	3	210	8	190	2	170	1
249	2	229	1	209	9	189	1	169	1
248	1	228	0	208	1	188	2	168	0
247	1	227	2	207	9	187	1	167	0
246	0	226	3	206	8	186	0	166	0
245	1	225	3	205	6	185	2	165	1
244	2	224	2	204	8	184	1	164	0
243	3	223	1	203	4	183	1	163	0
242	2	222	2	202	5	182	1	162	0
241	1	221	1	201	4	181	1	161	1

Graphical presentations of frequency distributions

Frequency distributions are often presented as graphs, most commonly as **histograms.** Figure 1–1 is a histogram of the grouped frequency distribution shown in Table 1–2; the **abscissa** (X or horizontal axis) shows the grouped scores, and the **ordinate** (Y or vertical axis) shows the frequencies.

To display nominal scale data, a **bar graph** is typically used. For example, if a group of 100 men had a mean serum cholesterol value of 212 mg/dl, and a group of 100 women had a mean value of 185 mg/dl, the means of these two groups could be presented as a bar graph, as shown in Figure 1–2.

Bar graphs are identical to frequency histograms, except that each rectangle on the graph is clearly separated from the others by a space, showing that the data form separate categories (such as male and female) rather than continuous groups.

For ratio or interval scale data, a frequency distribution may be drawn as a **frequency polygon,** in which the midpoints of each class interval are joined by straight lines, as shown in Figure 1–3.

A cumulative frequency distribution can also be presented graphically as a polygon, as shown in Figure 1–4A. Cumulative frequency polygons typically form a characteristic S-shaped curve known as an **ogive,** which the curve in Figure 1–4A approximates.

Table 1-2

Interval	Frequency f	Relative f % rel f	Cumulative f % cum f
251–260	5	2.5	100.0
241–250	13	6.5	97.5
231–240	19	9.5	91.0
221–230	18	9.0	81.5
211–220	38	19.0	72.5
201–210	72	36.0	53.5
191–200	14	7.0	17.5
181–190	12	6.0	10.5
171–180	5	2.5	4.5
161–170	4	2.0	2.0

Centiles and other quantiles

The cumulative frequency polygon and the cumulative frequency distribution both illustrate the concept of **centile** (or **percentile**) **rank,** which states the percentage of observations that fall below any particular score. In the case of a grouped frequency distribution, such as the one in Table 1–2, centile ranks state the percentage of observations that fall within or below any given class interval. Centile ranks provide a way of giving information about one individual score in relation to all the other scores in a distribution.

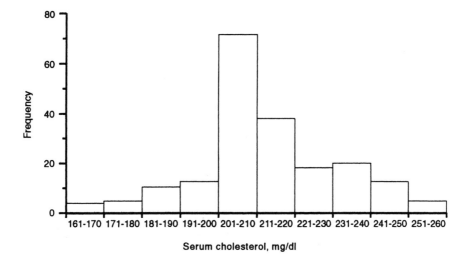

Figure 1-1

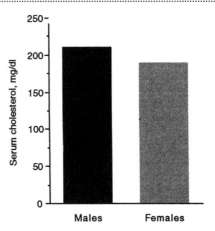

Figure 1-2

For example, the cumulative frequency column of Table 1–2 shows that 91% of the observations fall below 240.5 mg/dl, which therefore represents the 91st centile (which can be written as C_{91}), as shown in Figure 1–4B. A man with a serum cholesterol level of 240 mg/dl lies at the 91st centile—about 9% of the scores in the sample are higher than his.

Centile ranks are widely used in reporting scores on educational tests. They are one member of a family of values called **quantiles,** which divide distributions into a number of equal parts. Centiles divide a distribution into 100 equal parts. Other quantiles include **quartiles,** which divide the data into 4 parts, and **deciles,** which divide a distribution into 10 parts.

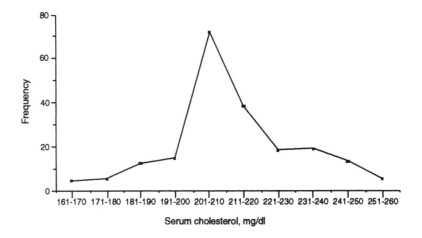

Figure 1-3

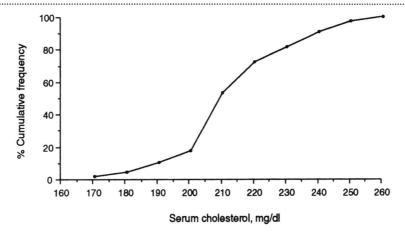

Figure 1-4A

The normal distribution

Frequency polygons may take many different shapes, but many naturally occurring phenomena are approximately distributed according to the symmetrical, bell-shaped **normal** or **Gaussian distribution,** as shown in Figure 1–5.

Skewed, J-shaped, and bimodal distributions

Figure 1–6 shows some other frequency distributions. Asymmetrical frequency distributions are called **skewed** distributions. **Positively** (or **right**) **skewed** distributions and **negatively** (or **left**) **skewed** distributions can be identified by the location of the *tail* of the curve (not by the location of the hump—

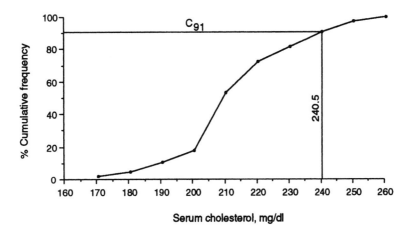

Figure 1-4B

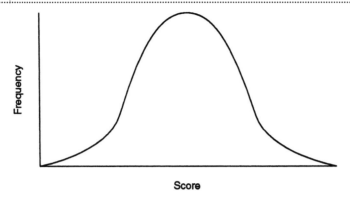

Figure 1-5

a common error). Positively skewed distributions have a relatively large number of low scores and a small number of very high scores, whereas negatively skewed distributions have a relatively large number of high scores and a small number of low scores.

Figure 1–6 also shows a **J-shaped** distribution and a **bimodal** distribution. Bimodal distributions are sometimes a combination of two underlying normal distributions, such as the heights of a large number of men and women—each gender forms its own normal distribution around a different midpoint.

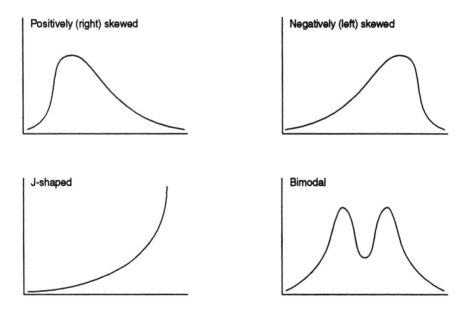

Figure 1-6

MEASURES OF CENTRAL TENDENCY

An entire distribution can be characterized by one typical measure that represents all the observations—**measures of central tendency.** These measures include the **mode,** the **median,** and the **mean.**

Mode
The mode is the observed value that occurs with the greatest frequency. It is found by simple inspection of the frequency distribution (it is easy to see on a frequency polygon as the highest point on the curve). If two scores both occur with the greatest frequency, the distribution is **bimodal;** if more than two scores occur with the greatest frequency, the distribution is multimodal. The mode is sometimes symbolized by **Mo.** *The mode is totally uninfluenced by small numbers of extreme scores in a distribution.*

Median
The median is the figure that divides the frequency distribution in half when all the scores are listed in order. When a distribution has an odd number of elements, the median is therefore the middle one; when it has an even number of elements, the median lies halfway between the two middle scores (i.e., it is the average or mean of the two middle scores).

For example, in a distribution consisting of the elements 6, 9, 15, 17, 24, the median would be 15. If the distribution were 6, 9, 15, 17, 24, 29, the median would be 16 (the average of 15 and 17).

The median responds only to the *number* of scores above it and below it, not to their actual values. If the above distribution were 6, 9, 15, 17, 24, 500 (rather than 29), the median would still be 16—so the median is *insensitive to small numbers of extreme scores in a distribution;* therefore, it is a very useful measure of central tendency for highly skewed distributions. The median is sometimes symbolized by **Mdn.** It is the same as the 50th centile (C_{50}).

Mean
The mean, or average, is the sum of all the elements divided by the number of elements in the distribution. It is symbolized by μ in a population, and by $\bar{X}$ ("x-bar") in a sample. The formulas for calculating the mean are therefore

$$\mu = \frac{\Sigma X}{N} \text{ in a population, and } \bar{X} = \frac{\Sigma X}{n} \text{ in a sample}$$

where Σ is "the sum of," so that $\Sigma X = X_1 + X_2 + X_3 + \ldots X_n$

Unlike other measures of central tendency, the mean responds to the *exact value* of every score in the distribution, and unlike the median and the mode, it is very sensitive to extreme scores. As a result, it is not usually an appropriate measure for characterizing very skewed distributions. On the other hand, it has a desirable property: repeated samples drawn from the same population will tend to have very similar means, and so the mean is the measure of central tendency that best resists the influence of fluctuation between different samples. For example, if repeated blood samples were taken from a patient, the mean number of white blood cells per high-powered microscope field would fluctuate less from sample to sample than would the modal or median number of cells.

The relationship among the three measures of central tendency depends on the shape of the distribution. In a unimodal symmetrical distribution (such as the normal distribution), all three measures are identical, but in a skewed distribution they will usually differ. Figures 1–7 and 1–8 show positively and negatively skewed distributions, respectively. In both of these, the mode is simply the most frequently occurring score (the highest point on the curve); the mean is pulled up or down by the influence of a relatively small number of very high or very low scores; and the median lies between the two, dividing the distribution into two equal areas under the curve.

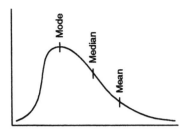

Figure 1-7

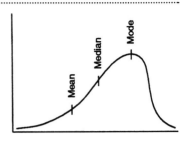

Figure 1-8

MEASURES OF VARIABILITY

Figure 1–9 shows two normal distributions, A and B; their means, modes, and medians are all identical, and, like all normal distributions, they are symmetrical and unimodal. Despite these similarities, these two distributions are obviously different; therefore, describing a normal distribution in terms of the three measures of central tendency alone is clearly inadequate.

Although these two distributions have identical measures of central tendency, they differ in terms of their **variability**—the extent to which their scores are clustered together or scattered about. The scores forming distribution A are clearly more scattered than are those forming distribution B. Variability is a very important quality: if these two distributions represented the fasting glucose levels of diabetic patients taking two different drugs for glycemic control, for example, then drug B would be the better medication, as fewer patients on this distribution have very high or very low glucose levels—even though the *mean* effect of drug B is the same as that of drug A.

There are three important measures of variability: **range, variance,** and **standard deviation.**

Range

The range is the simplest measure of variability. It is the difference between the lowest and the highest scores in the distribution. It therefore responds to these two scores only.

> For example, in the distribution 6, 9, 15, 17, 24, the range is $(24 - 6) = 18$; but in the distribution 6, 9, 15, 17, 24, 500, the range is $(500 - 6) = 494$.

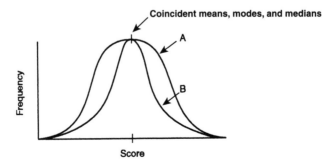

Figure 1-9

Variance (and deviation scores)   Calculating variance (and standard deviation) involves the use of **deviation scores.** The deviation score of an element is found by subtracting the distribution's mean from the element. A deviation score is symbolized by the letter *x* (as opposed to X, which symbolizes an element); so the formula for deviation scores is

$$x = X - \bar{x}$$

For example, in a distribution with a mean of 16, an element of 23 would have a deviation score of $(23 - 16) = 7$. On the same distribution, an element of 11 would have a deviation score of $(11 - 16) = -5$.

When calculating deviation scores for all the elements in a distribution, the results can be verified by checking that the sum of the deviation scores for all the elements is zero; i.e., $\Sigma\, x = 0$.

The **variance** of a distribution is the mean of the squares of all the deviation scores in the distribution. The variance is therefore obtained by:

- finding the deviation score (x) for each element,

- squaring each of these deviation scores (thus eliminating minus signs), and then

- obtaining their mean in the usual way—by adding them all up and then dividing the total by their number.

Variance is symbolized by σ^2 for a population and by S^2 for a sample. Thus,

$$\sigma^2 = \frac{\Sigma(X - \mu)^2}{N} \text{ or } \frac{\Sigma x^2}{N} \text{ in a population, and } S^2 = \frac{\Sigma (X - \bar{X})^2}{n} \text{ or } \frac{\Sigma x^2}{n} \text{ in a sample.}[1]$$

Variance is sometimes known as **mean square.** Variance is expressed in squared units of measurement, limiting its usefulness as a descriptive term—its intuitive meaning is poor.

Standard deviation   The standard deviation remedies this problem: it is the *square root* of the variance, so it is expressed in the same units of measurement as the original data. The symbols for standard deviation are therefore the same as the symbols for variance, but without being raised to the power of two. So the standard deviation of a population is σ, and the standard deviation of a sample is **S.** Standard deviation is sometimes written as **SD.**

The standard deviation is particularly useful in normal distributions, because *the proportion of elements in the normal distribution* (i.e., the proportion of the area under the curve) *is a constant for a given number of standard deviations above or below the mean of the distribution,* as shown in Figure 1–10.

In Figure 1–10:

- approximately **68%** of the distribution falls within ±**1** standard deviation of the mean,

- approximately **95%** of the distribution falls within ±**2** standard deviations of the mean,

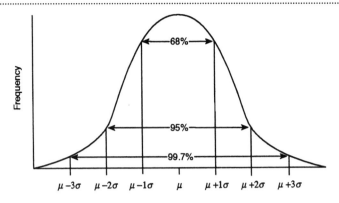

Figure 1-10

- and approximately **99.7%** of the distribution falls within ±3 standard deviations of the mean.

---

*Because these proportions hold true for **every** normal distribution, they should be memorized.*

Therefore, if a population's resting heart rate is normally distributed with a mean (μ) of 70 and a standard deviation (S) of 10, the proportion of the population that has a resting heart rate between certain limits can be stated.

As Figure 1–11 shows, because 68% of the distribution lies within approximately ±1 standard deviations of the mean, 68% of the population will have a resting heart rate between 60 and 80 beats/min.

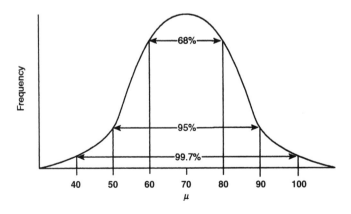

Figure 1-11

Similarly, 95% of the population will have a heart rate between approximately $70 \pm (2 \times 10) = 50$ and 90 beats/min (i.e., within 2 standard deviations of the mean).

Z SCORES

The location of any element in a normal distribution can be expressed in terms of how many standard deviations it lies above or below the mean of the distribution. This is the *z score* of the element. If the element lies above the mean, it will have a positive *z* score; if it lies below the mean, it will have a negative *z* score.

For example, a heart rate of 85 beats/min in the distribution shown in Figure 1–11 lies 1.5 standard deviations above the mean, so it has a *z* score of +1.5. A heart rate of 65 lies 0.5 standard deviations below the mean, so its *z* score is −0.5. The formula for calculating *z* scores is therefore

$$z = \frac{X - \mu}{\sigma}$$

Tables of *z* scores

Tables of *z* scores state what proportion of any normal distribution lies above *any* given *z* scores, not just *z* scores of ±1, 2, or 3.

Table 1–3 is an abbreviated table of *z* scores; it shows, for example, that .3085 (or about 31%) of any normal distribution lies above a *z* score of +0.5. Because normal distributions are symmetrical, this also means that approximately 31% of the distribution lies *below* a *z* score of −0.5 (which corresponds to a heart rate of 65 beats/min in Fig. 1–11)—so approximately 31% of this population has a heart rate below 65 beats/min. By subtracting this proportion from 1, it is apparent that .6915, or about 69%, of the population has a heart rate of *above* 65 beats/min.

Z scores are standardized or normalized, so they allow scores on different normal distributions to be compared. For example, a person's height could be compared with his or her weight by means of the respective *z* scores (provided that both these variables are elements in normal distributions).

Instead of using *z* scores to find the proportion of a distribution corresponding to a particular score, we can also do the converse: use *z* scores to find the score that divides the distribution into specified proportions.

> For example, if we want to know what heart rate divides the fastest-beating 5% of the population (i.e., the group at or above the 95th percentile) from the remaining 95%, we can use the *z* score table.

In this instance, we want to find the *z* score that divides the top 5% of the area under the curve from the remaining area. In Table 1–3, the nearest figure to 5% (.05) is .0495; the *z* score corresponding to this is 1.65.

As Figure 1–12 shows, the corresponding heart rate therefore lies 1.65 standard deviations above the mean, i.e., it is equal to $\mu + 1.65\sigma = 70 + (1.65 \times 10) = 86.5$. We can conclude that the fastest-beating 5% of this population has a heart rate above 86.5 beats/min.

The *z* score that divides the top 5% of the population from the remaining 95% is *not* approximately 2. Although 95% of the distribution falls between approximately ±2 standard deviations of the mean, this is the *middle* 95% (see Fig. 1–11). This leaves the remaining 5% split into two equal parts at the two tails of the distribution (remember—normal distributions are symmetrical). Therefore, only 2.5% of the distribution falls more than 2 standard deviations *above* the mean, and another 2.5% falls more than 2 standard deviations *below* the mean.

Table 1-3

z	Area beyond z	z	Area beyond z
0.00	.5000	1.65	.0495
0.05	.4801	1.70	.0446
0.10	.4602	1.75	.0401
0.15	.4404	1.80	.0359
0.20	.4207	1.85	.0322
0.25	.4013	1.90	.0287
0.30	.3821	1.95	.0256
0.35	.3632	2.00	.0228
0.40	.3446	2.05	.0202
0.45	.3264	2.10	.0179
0.50	.3085	2.15	.0158
0.55	.2912	2.20	.0139
0.60	.2743	2.25	.0112
0.65	.2578	2.30	.0107
0.70	.2420	2.35	.0094
0.75	.2266	2.40	.0082
0.80	.2119	2.45	.0071
0.85	.1977	2.50	.0062
0.90	.1841	2.55	.0054
0.95	.1711	2.60	.0047
1.00	.1587	2.65	.0040
1.05	.1469	2.70	.0035
1.10	.1357	2.75	.0030
1.15	.1251	2.80	.0026
1.20	.1151	2.85	.0022
1.25	.1056	2.90	.0019
1.30	.0968	2.95	.0016
1.35	.0885	3.00	.0013
1.40	.0808	3.05	.0011
1.45	.0735	3.10	.0010
1.50	.0668	3.15	.0008
1.55	.0606	3.20	.0007
1.60	.0548	3.30	.0005

This table is not a complete listing of z scores. Full z score tables can be found in most statistics textbooks.

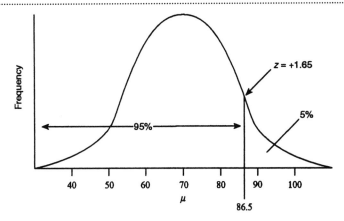

Figure 1-12

Using *z* scores to specify probability

Z scores also allow us to specify the probability of a randomly picked element being above or below a particular score.

> For example, if we know that 5% of the population has a heart rate above 86.5 beats/min, then the probability of one randomly selected person from this population having a heart rate above 86.5 beats/min will be 5%, or .05.

We can find the probability that a random person will have a pulse less than 50 beats/min in the same way. Because 50 lies 2 standard deviations (i.e., 2×10) below the mean (70), it corresponds to a z score of -2, and we know that approximately 95% of the distribution lies within the limits $z = \pm2$. Therefore, 5% of the distribution lies outside these limits, equally in each of the two tails of the distribution. So 2.5% of the distribution lies below 50, and the probability that a randomly selected person has a pulse less than 50 beats/min is 2.5%, or .025.

NOTE

[1]Some statisticians prefer to use a denominator of $n - 1$ rather than n in the formula for sample variance. Both formulas are correct; using $n - 1$ is preferred when the variance of a small sample is being used to estimate the variance of the population.

EXERCISES

Select the **single best answer** to the questions referring to the following scenario.

A family physician is interested in the cigarette use of patients in her practice. She asks all patients who come into her office if they use cigarettes and determines that 20% of her patients smoke. She then asks every third smoker who comes to the office how many cigarettes they smoke each day; she finds that the mean number of cigarettes smoked is 16. She plots the number of cigarettes smoked by each patient on a frequency distribution and finds that it is normally distributed. She also finds that the number of male smokers is equal to the number of female smokers. She already knows that half of her patients are men, and half are women.

1. Which of the following characteristics of the sample taken by the physician in the above scenario would cause the sample to be biased?

a. The fact that the number of cigarettes smoked is normally distributed.
b. The fact that systematic samples cannot be representative.
c. The fact that the number of male smokers is equal to the number of female smokers.
d. The fact that smokers who come to the office are more likely to be sick, and perhaps more likely to smoke more cigarettes, than smokers who do not come to the office.

2. How likely is it that two patients who smoke will independently appear in succession in the physician's office?

a. .20
b. .40
c. .02
d. .04
e. .016

3. How likely is it that the next patient to come to the office will be a woman or a smoker?

a. .7
b. .20
c. .04
d. .07
e. .02

4. What type of data is formed by the figures the physician has generated regarding the number of cigarettes her patients smoke?

a. Nominal
b. Ordinal
c. Interval
d. Ratio
e. Continuous

5. On the frequency distribution showing the number of cigarettes smoked, what is the relationship between the three measures of central tendency?

a. The mean, mode, and median will all be at the same point.
b. The mean will be lower than the median, which will be lower than the mode.
c. The mean will be higher than the median, which will be higher than the mode.
d. It is impossible to say from the information given.

6. A particular patient, Mr. A., smokes 24 cigarettes a day. What is the corresponding deviation score?

a. 24
b. 40
c. 0
d. +8
e. −8

7. The physician determines the deviation scores for each smoking patient in her sample, squares each of these scores, adds up all the squared scores, and then divides them by the number of smoking patients in her sample. The resulting figure is

   a. the range.
   b. the percentile rank.
   c. the variance.
   d. the standard deviation.

8. If she finds that the variance of the number of cigarettes smoked is 16, what is the standard deviation?

   a. 20
   b. 36
   c. 16
   d. 4
   e. 0

9. What is the z score corresponding to the number of cigarettes (24) smoked by Mr. A.?

   a. -2
   b. $+2$
   c. 0
   d. $+8$
   e. -8

10. Assuming the physician's sample of smokers is representative of all the smokers in her practice, what proportion of smokers smoke more than 24 cigarettes a day?

   a. 2.5%
   b. 5%
   c. 7.5%
   d. 16%
   e. 24%

11. Assuming the physician's sample of smokers is representative of all the smokers in her practice, what proportion of smokers smoke more than 20 cigarettes a day?

   a. 2.5%
   b. 5%
   c. 7.5%
   d. 16%
   e. 24%

12. Assuming the physician's sample of smokers is representative of all the smokers in her practice, how likely is it that the next smoker who comes to the office smokes less than 12 cigarettes per day? (Use the standard deviation calculated in Question 8).

a. 2.5%
b. 5%
c. 7.5%
d. 16%
e. 24%

13. Approximately how many cigarettes would a smoker have to smoke each day to lie at the 95th percentile of smokers in this physician's practice? (Refer to Table 1–3).

a. 16
b. 18
c. 23
d. 24
e. 32

2

Inferential Statistics

At the end of the previous chapter, it was shown how z scores can be used to find the probability that a random element will have a score above or below a certain value. To do this, the population had to be normally distributed, and both the population mean (μ) and the population standard deviation (σ) had to be known.

Most research, however, involves the opposite kind of problem: instead of using information about a *population* to draw conclusions or make predictions about a *sample*, the researcher usually wants to use the information provided by a *sample* to draw conclusions about a *population*. For example, a researcher might want to forecast the results of an election on the basis of an opinion poll, or predict the effectiveness of a new drug for all patients with a particular disease after it has been tested on only a small sample of patients.

STATISTICS AND PARAMETERS

In such problems, the population mean and standard deviation, μ and σ (which are called the population **parameters**), are unknown; all that is known is the sample mean ($\overline{X}$) and standard deviation (S)—these are called the sample **statistics.** The task of using a sample to draw conclusions about a population involves going beyond the actual information that is available; in other words, it involves **inference.** Inferential statistics therefore involve using a statistic to estimate a parameter.

However, it is unlikely that a sample will perfectly represent the population it is drawn from: a statistic (such as the sample mean) will not exactly reflect its corresponding parameter (the population mean). For example, in a study of intelligence, if a sample of 1000 people is drawn from a population with a mean IQ of 100, it would not be expected that the mean IQ of the sample would be *exactly* 100. There will be **sampling error**—which is not an error, but just natural, expected random variation—that will cause the sample statistic to differ from the population parameter. Similarly, if a coin is tossed 1000 times, even if it is perfectly fair, getting *exactly* 500 heads and 500 tails would not be expected.

The random sampling distribution of means

Imagine you have a hat containing 100 pieces of paper, numbered from zero to 99. At random, you take out five pieces of paper, record the number written on each one, and find the mean of these five numbers. Then you put the pieces of paper back in the hat and draw another random sample, repeating the same process for approximately 10 minutes.

Do you expect that the means of each of these samples will be exactly the same? Of course not. Because of sampling error, they vary somewhat. If you plot all the means on a frequency distribution, the sample means form a distribution, called the **random sampling distribution of means.**

If you actually try this, you will note that this distribution looks pretty much like a normal distribution. If you continued drawing samples and plotting their means *ad infinitum*, you would find that the distribution actually becomes a normal distribution! This holds true even if the underlying population was not at all normally distributed: in our population of pieces of paper in the hat, there is just one piece of paper with each number, so the shape of the distribution is actually *rectangular*, as shown in Figure 2–1, yet its random sampling distribution of means still tends to be normal.

These principles are stated by a theorem, called the **central limit theorem,** which states that the *random sampling distribution of means will always tend to be normal, irrespective of the shape of the population distribution from which the samples were drawn*. Figure 2–2 is a random sampling distribution of means; even if the underlying population formed a rectangular, skewed, or any other non-normal distribution, the means of all the random samples drawn from it will always tend to form a normal distribution. The theorem further states that the random sampling distribution of means will become closer to normal as the size of the samples increases.

The theorem also states that the mean of the random sampling distribution of means (symbolized by $\mu_{\bar{x}}$, showing that it is the mean of the population of all the sample means) is equal to the mean of the original population; in other words, $\mu_{\bar{x}}$ is equal to μ. (If Figure 2–2 was superimposed on Figure 2–1, the means would be the same).

Like all distributions, the random sampling distribution of means shown in Figure 2–2 not only has a mean, but it also has a standard deviation. As always, standard deviation is a measure of variability—a measure of the degree to which the elements of the distribution are clustered together or scattered widely apart. This particular standard deviation, the standard deviation of the random sampling distribution of means, is symbolized by $\sigma_{\bar{x}}$, signifying that it is the standard deviation of the population of all the sample means. It has its own name: **standard error,** or **standard error of the mean,** sometimes abbreviated as *SE* or *SEM*. It is a measure of the extent to which the sample means deviate from the true population mean.

Figure 2–2 shows the obvious: when repeated random samples are drawn from a population, most of the means of those samples are going to cluster around the original population mean. In the "numbers in the hat" example, one would expect to find many sample means clustering around 50 (between 40 and 60). Rather fewer sample means would fall between 30 and 40 or between 60 and 70. Far fewer would lie out toward the extreme "tails" of the distribution (between 0 and 20 or between 80 and 99).

If the sample consisted of just two pieces of paper, what would happen to the shape of Figure 2–2? Clearly, with an *n* of just 2, the sample means would be quite likely to lie out toward the tails of the distribution, giving a broader, fatter shape to the curve, and hence a higher standard error. On the

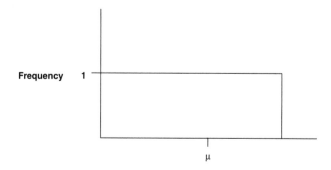

Figure 2-1

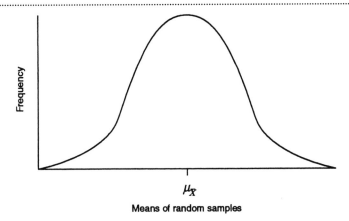

Frequency

$\mu_{\overline{x}}$

Means of random samples

Figure 2-2   The random sampling distribution of means: the ultimate result of drawing a large number of random samples from a population and plotting each of their individual means on a frequency distribution.

other hand, if the sample consisted of 25 pieces of paper ($n = 25$), it would be very unlikely for many of their means to lie far from the center of the curve. Therefore, there would be a much thinner, narrower curve and a lower standard error.

Thus, the shape of the random sampling distribution of means, as reflected by its standard error, is affected by the size of the samples. In fact, the standard error is equal to the population standard deviation (σ) divided by the square root of the size of the samples (n). Therefore, the formula for the standard error is

$$\sigma_{\overline{x}} = \frac{\sigma}{\sqrt{n}}$$

Standard error

As the formula shows, the standard error is dependent on the size of the samples: *standard error is inversely related to the square root of the sample size*, so that the larger n becomes, the more closely will the sample means represent the true population mean. *This is the mathematical reason why the results of large studies or surveys are more trusted than the results of small ones*—a fact that is intuitively obvious!

Predicting the probability of drawing samples with a given mean

Because the random sampling distribution of means is by definition normal, the known facts about normal distributions and z scores can be used to find the probability that a *sample* will have a *mean* of above or below a given value, provided, of course, that the sample is a random one. This is a step beyond what was possible in Chapter 1, where only the probability that *one element* would have a score above or below a given value was predicted.

In addition, because the random sampling distribution of means is normal even when the underlying population is not normally distributed, z scores can be used to make predictions, regardless of the underlying population distribution—provided, once again, that the sample is random.

Using the standard error

The method used to make a prediction about a sample mean is similar to the method used in Chapter 1 to make a prediction about a single element—it involves finding the z score corresponding to the value of interest. However, instead of calculating the z score in terms of the number of *standard deviations* by which a given *single element* lies above or below the population mean, the z score is now calculated in terms of the number of *standard errors* by which a *sample mean* lies above or below the population mean. Therefore, the previous formula

$$z = \frac{X - \mu}{\sigma} \quad \text{now becomes} \quad z = \frac{\bar{X} - \mu}{\sigma_{\bar{x}}}$$

For example, in a population with a mean resting heart rate of 70 beats/min and a standard deviation of 10, the probability that a random sample of 25 people will have a mean heart rate above 75 beats/min can be determined. The steps are:

1. Calculate the standard error: $\sigma_{\bar{x}} = \dfrac{\sigma}{\sqrt{n}} = \dfrac{10}{\sqrt{25}} = 2$

2. Calculate the z score of the sample mean: $z = \dfrac{\bar{X} - \mu}{\sigma_{\bar{x}}} = \dfrac{75 - 70}{2} = 2.5$

3. Find the proportion of the normal distribution that lies beyond this z score (2.5). Table 1–3 shows that this proportion is .0062. Therefore, the probability that a random sample of 25 people from this population will have a mean resting heart rate above 75 beats/min is .0062.

Conversely, it is possible to find what random sample mean ($n = 25$) is so high that it would occur in only 5% or less of all samples (in other words, what mean is so high that the probability of obtaining it is .05 or less):

Table 1–3 shows that the z score that divides the bottom 95% of the distribution from the top 5% is 1.65. The corresponding heart rate is $\mu + 1.65\,\sigma_{\bar{x}}$ (the population mean plus 1.65 standard errors). As the population mean is 70 and the standard error is 2, the heart rate will be 70 + (1.65 ×2), or 73.3. Figure 2–3 shows the relevant portions of the random sampling distribu-

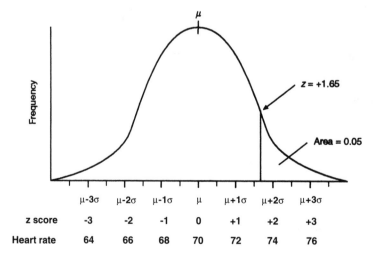

Figure 2-3

tion of means; the appropriate z score is $+1.65$, not $+2$, because it refers to the *top .05* of the distribution, not the top .025 and the bottom .025 together.

It is also possible to find the limits between which 95% of all possible random sample means would be expected to fall. As with any normal distribution, 95% of the random sampling distribution of means lie within approximately ± 2 standard errors of the population mean (in other words, within $z = \pm 2$); therefore, 95% of all possible sample means must lie within approximately ± 2 standard errors of the population mean. [As Table 1–3 shows, the *exact* z scores that correspond to the middle 95% of any normal distribution are in fact ± 1.96, not ± 2; the exact limits are therefore $70 \pm (1.96 \times 2) = 66.08$ and 73.92]. Applying this to the distribution of resting heart rate, it is apparent that 95% of all possible random sample means will fall between the limits of $\mu \pm 2\,\sigma_{\bar{x}}$, that is, approximately $70 \pm (2 \times 2)$, or 66 and 74.

ESTIMATING THE MEAN OF A POPULATION

So far it has been shown how z scores are used to find the probability that a random sample will have a mean of above or below a given value. It has been shown that 95% of all possible members of the population will lie within approximately ± 2 (or, more exactly, ± 1.96) standard errors of the population mean, and 95% of all such means will be within ± 2 standard errors of the mean.

Confidence limits

Logically, if the sample mean ($\bar{X}$) lies within ± 1.96 standard errors of the population mean (μ) 95% (.95) of the time, then μ must lie within ± 1.96 standard errors of $\bar{X}$ 95% of the time. These limits of ± 1.96 standard errors are called the **confidence limits** (in this case, the 95% confidence limits). Finding the confidence limits involves inferential statistics, because a sample statistic ($\bar{X}$) is being used to estimate a population parameter (μ).

For example, if a researcher wishes to find the true mean resting heart rate of a large population, it would be impractical to take the pulse of every person in the population. Instead, he or she would draw a random sample from the population and take the pulse of the persons in the sample. As long as the sample is truly random, the researcher can be 95% confident that the true population mean lies within ± 1.96 standard errors of the sample mean.

Therefore, if the mean heart rate of the sample ($\bar{X}$) is 74 and $\sigma_{\bar{x}} = 2$, the researcher can be 95% certain that μ lies within 1.96 standard errors of 74, i.e., between $74 \pm (1.96 \times 2)$, or 70.08 and 77.92. The best *single* estimate of the population mean is still the sample mean, 74—after all, it is the only piece of actual data on which an estimate can be based.

In general, confidence limits are equal to the sample mean plus or minus the z score obtained from the table (for the appropriate level of confidence) multiplied by the standard error:

$$\text{Confidence limits} = \bar{X} \pm z\,\sigma_{\bar{x}}$$

Therefore, 95% confidence limits (which are the ones conventionally used in medical research) are approximately equal to the sample mean plus or minus two standard errors.

The difference between the upper and lower confidence limits is called the **confidence interval**—sometimes abbreviated as *CI*.

Researchers obviously want the confidence interval to be as narrow as possible. The formula for confidence limits shows that to make the confidence interval narrower (for a given level of confidence, such as 95%) the standard error ($\sigma_{\bar{x}}$) must be made smaller. Standard error is found by the formula $\sigma_{\bar{x}} = \sigma \div \sqrt{n}$. Because σ is a population parameter that the researcher cannot change, the only way to reduce standard error is to increase the sample size n. Once again, there is a mathematical reason why large studies are trusted more than small ones. Note that the formula for standard error means that standard error will decrease only in proportion to the *square root* of the sample size; therefore, the width of the confidence interval will decrease in proportion to the square root of the sample size. In other words, to *halve* the confidence interval, the sample size must be increased *fourfold*.

Precision and accuracy

Precision is the degree to which a figure (such as an estimate of a population mean) is immune from random variation. The width of the confidence interval reflects precision—the wider the confidence interval, the less precise the estimate.

Because the width of the confidence interval decreases in proportion to the square root of sample size, *precision is proportional to the square root of sample size*. To double the precision of an estimate, sample size must be multiplied by 4; to triple precision, sample size must be multiplied by 9; and to quadruple precision, sample size must be multiplied by 16. Increasing the precision of research therefore requires disproportionate increases in sample size; thus, very precise research is expensive and time-consuming.

Precision must be distinguished from **accuracy,** which is the degree to which an estimate is immune from systematic error or bias.

A good way to remember the difference between precision and accuracy is to think of a person playing darts, aiming at the bull's eye in the center of the dartboard. Figure 2–4A shows how the dartboard looks after a player has thrown five darts. Is there much systematic error (bias)? No. The darts do not tend to err in any one direction. However, although there is no bias, there is much random variation, as the darts are not clustered together. Hence, the player's aim is **unbiased** (or **accurate**) but imprecise. It may seem strange to call such a poor player accurate, but the darts are at least centered on the bull's eye, on average. The player needs to reduce the random variation in his or her aim, rather than aim at a different point.

Figure 2–4B shows a different scenario, but the same questions can be asked. Is there much systematic error or bias? Certainly. The player consistently throws toward the top left of the dartboard, and so the aim is **biased** (or **inaccurate**). Is there much random variation? No. The darts are tightly clustered together, hence relatively immune from random variation. The player's aim is therefore **precise.**

Figure 2–4C shows darts that are not only widely scattered, but also systematically err in one direction. Thus, this player's aim is not immune from either bias or random variation, making it **biased** (**inaccurate**) and **imprecise.**

Figure 2–4D shows the ideal, both in darts and in inferential statistics. There is no systematic error or significant random variation, so this aim is both **accurate** (**unbiased**) and **precise.**

Figure 2–5 shows the same principles in terms of four hypothetical random sampling distributions of means. Each curve shows the result of taking a very large number of samples from the same population and then plotting their means on a frequency distribution. **Precision** is shown by the narrowness of each curve: as in all frequency distributions, the spread of the distribution around its mean reflects its variability. A very spread-out curve has a high variability and a high standard error and therefore provides an imprecise estimate of the true population mean. **Accuracy** is shown by the distance between the mean of the random sampling distribution of means ($\mu_{\bar{x}}$) and the true population mean (μ). This is analogous to a darts player with an inaccurate aim and a considerable distance between the average position of his or her darts and the bull's eye.

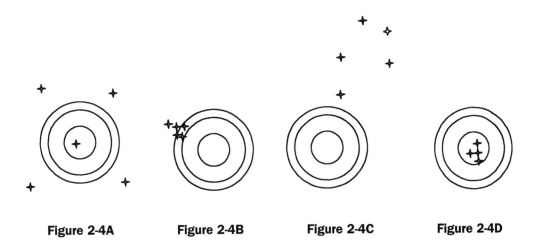

Figure 2-4A   **Figure 2-4B**   **Figure 2-4C**   **Figure 2-4D**

Distribution A in Figure 2–5 is a very spread-out random sampling distribution of means; thus, it provides an **imprecise** estimate of the true population mean. However, its mean does coincide with the true population mean, and so it provides an **accurate** estimate of the true population mean. In other words, the estimate that it provides is not biased, but it is subject to considerable random variation. This is the type of result that would occur if the samples were truly random but small.

Distribution B is a narrow distribution, which therefore provides a **precise** estimate of the true population mean. Due to the low standard error, the width of the confidence interval would be narrow. However, its mean lies a long way from the true population mean, so it will provide a **biased** estimate

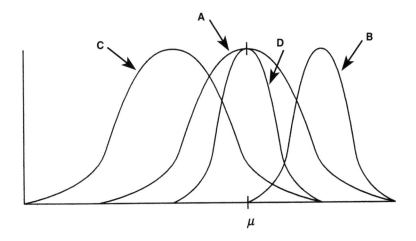

Figure 2-5

of the true population mean. This is the kind of result that is produced by large but biased (i.e., not truly random) samples.

Distribution C has the worst of both worlds: it is very spread out (having a high standard error) and would therefore provide an **imprecise** estimate of the true population mean. Its mean lies a long way from the true population mean, so its estimate is also **biased.** This would occur if the samples were small and biased.

Distribution D is narrow, and therefore precise, and its mean lies at the same point as the true population mean, so it is also **accurate.** This ideal is the kind of distribution that would be obtained from large and truly random samples; therefore, to achieve maximum precision and accuracy in inferential statistics, samples should be large and truly random.

Estimating the standard error

So far it has been shown how to determine the probability that a random sample will have a mean that is above or below a certain value, and it has been shown how the mean of a sample can be used to estimate the mean of the population from which it was drawn, with a known degree of precision and confidence. All this has been done by using z scores, which express the number of standard errors by which a sample mean lies above or below the true population mean.

However, because standard error is found from the formula $\sigma_{\bar{x}} = \sigma \div \sqrt{n}$, we cannot calculate standard error unless we know σ, the population standard deviation. In practice, however, σ will not be known; researchers hardly ever know the standard deviation of the population (and if they did, they would probably not need to use inferential statistics anyway).

As a result, standard error cannot be calculated, and therefore z scores cannot be used. Instead, the standard error can be *estimated* using data that *are* available from the sample alone. The resulting statistic is the **estimated standard error of the mean,** usually called estimated standard error (although, confusingly, it is called standard error in many research articles); it is symbolized by $s_{\bar{x}}$, and it is found by the formula

Estimated standard error of the mean

$$s_{\bar{x}} = \frac{S}{\sqrt{n-1}}$$

where S is the sample standard deviation, as defined in Chapter 1.

t scores

The estimated standard error is used to find a statistic, called t, that can be used in place of z. The t score, rather than the z score, *must* be used when making inferences about means that are based on *estimates* of population parameters (such as estimated standard error) rather than on the population parameters themselves. The t score is sometimes known as the **Student's t.** (Its inventor was employed by Guinness breweries to perform quality control on the beer. Because of this situation, he could not name the statistic after himself, but gave himself the pseudonym "Student.")

The t score is calculated in much the same way as z. However, whereas z was expressed in terms of the number of standard errors by which a sample mean lies above or below the population mean, t is expressed in terms of the number of *estimated* standard errors by which the sample mean lies above or below the population mean. The formula for t is therefore

$$t = \frac{\bar{X} - \mu}{s_{\bar{x}}}$$

Compare this formula with the formula we used for z:

$$z = \frac{\overline{X} - \mu}{\sigma_{\overline{x}}}$$

Just as z score tables give the proportions of the normal distribution that lie above and below any given z score, so there are t score tables that provide the same information for any given t score. However, there is one difference between these tables. Whereas the value of z for any given proportion of the distribution is constant (e.g., z values of ±1.96 *always* delineate the middle 95% of the distribution), the value of t for any given proportion is not constant—it varies from one sample to the next. When the sample size is large ($n > 100$), the values of t and z are similar. As samples get smaller, t and z scores become increasingly different.

Degrees of freedom and *t* tables

Table 2–1 is an abbreviated t score table that shows the values of t corresponding to different areas under the normal distribution for various sample sizes. Tables of t values do not show sample size (n) directly; instead, they express sample size in terms of degrees of freedom (df). For the purposes of USMLE, degrees of freedom (df) can be defined as simply equal to $n - 1$. Therefore, to determine the value of t (such that 95% of the population of t-statistics based on a sample size of 15 lies between $-t$ and $+t$), one would look in the table for the appropriate value of t for $df = 14$ (14 being equal to n $- 1$); this is sometimes written as t_{14}. Table 2–1 shows that this value is 2.145.

As n becomes larger (100 or more), the values of t are very close to the corresponding values of z. As the middle column shows, for a df of 100, 95% of the distribution falls within $t = \pm1.984$; while for a df of ∞ this figure is 1.96, which is the same figure for z (see Table 1–3). In general, the value of t that divides the central 95% of the distribution from the remaining 5% is in the region of 2, just as it is for z. (One- and two-tailed tests are discussed in Chapter 3 in the section on Directional Hypotheses).

As an example of the use of t scores, we can repear the earlier task of estimating (with 95% confidence) the true mean resting heart rate of a large population, basing the estimate on a random sample of people drawn from this population. This time we will not make the unrealistic assumption that the standard error is known.

As before, a random sample of 15 people is drawn, and it is found that their mean heart rate ($\overline{X}$) is 74 beats/min. Assuming that the standard deviation of this sample is 8.2, the estimated standard error, $\sigma_{\overline{X}}$, can be calculated as follows:

$$s_{\overline{x}} = \frac{S}{\sqrt{n - 1}}$$
$$= \frac{8.2}{\sqrt{15 - 1}}$$
$$= \frac{8.2}{3.74}$$
$$= 2.2$$

For a sample consisting of 15 people, the t tables will give the appropriate value of t (corresponding to the middle 95% of the distribution) for $df = 14$ (i.e., n $- 1$).

Table 2–1 shows that this value is 2.145. This value is not very different from the "ballpark" 95% figure for z, which is 2. The 95% confidence intervals are therefore equal to the sample mean plus or minus t times the estimated standard error (i.e., $\overline{X} \pm t \times s_{\overline{X}}$), which in this example is

Table 2-1

Area in 2 tails	.100	.050	.010	
Area in 1 tail	.050	.025	.005	
df				
1	6.314	12.706	63.657	
2	2.920	4.303	9.925	
3	2.353	3.182	5.841	
4	2.132	2.776	4.604	
5	2.015	2.571	4.032	
6	1.943	2.447	3.707	
7	1.895	2.365	3.499	
8	1.860	2.306	3.355	
9	1.833	2.262	3.250	
10	1.812	2.228	3.169	
11	1.796	2.201	3.106	
12	1.782	2.179	3.055	
13	1.771	2.160	3.012	
14	1.761	2.145	2.977	
15	1.753	2.131	2.947	
25	1.708	2.060	2.787	
50	1.676	2.009	2.678	
100	1.660	1.984	2.626	
∞+	1.645	1.960	2.576	

This table is not a complete listing of *t*-statistics values. Full tables may be found in most statistics textbooks.

$$74 \pm (2.145 \times 2.2) = 69.281 \text{ and } 78.719.$$

The sample mean therefore allows for the estimate that the true mean resting heart rate of this population is 74 beats/min. One can be 95% confident that it lies between 69.281 and 78.719.

Because the figure for *t* for 95% confidence intervals is almost invariably going to be in the region of 2 (Table 2–1), it should be noted that in general, *one can be 95% confident that the true mean of a population lies within approximately plus or minus two estimated standard errors of the mean of a random sample drawn from that population.*

EXERCISES

Select the **single best answer** to the following questions, referring to the appropriate scenarios.

Questions 1–8

A researcher is interested in comparing the rates of obesity in different cities. He wants to start by finding the mean weight of adult male New Yorkers.

1.   You would advise him to

a.   start by trying to verify that adult male New Yorkers' weights are normally distributed.
b.   weigh every adult male New Yorker and calculate their mean weight.
c.   draw a nonrandom sample of 1000 adult male New Yorkers, weigh them, and calculate the mean weight of the sample.
d.   draw a random sample of 10 adult male New Yorkers, weigh them, and calculate the mean weight of the sample.
e.   draw a random sample of 500 adult male New Yorkers, weigh them, and calculate the mean weight of the sample.

2.   Which of the following sampling plans is most likely to give an accurate but imprecise estimate of the weight of adult male New Yorkers?

a.   Weighing 5000 people randomly selected from a list of adult male registered voters in New York.
b.   Weighing 100 people randomly selected from a list of adult male registered voters in New York.
c.   Weighing 5000 people who were randomly selected from adult males jogging in Central Park.
d.   Weighing 100 people who were randomly selected from adult males jogging in Central Park.

3.   The researcher draws an unbiased sample of 101 adult male New Yorkers. Their mean weight is 72 kg, and the standard deviation is 15. The estimated standard error is therefore

a.   impossible to calculate with the information given.
b.   150.
c.   1.5.
d.   square root of 1.
e.   72/15.

4.   If the estimated standard error is 1.5, the researcher can state that he is 95% confident that the true mean weight of all adult male New Yorkers lies between

a.   66 and 78 kg.
b.   69 and 75 kg.
c.   70.5 and 73.5 kg.
d.   None of the above.

5.   The width of the 95% confidence interval of the researcher's estimate is

a.   12 kg.
b.   6 kg.

c. 3 kg.
d. None of the above.

6. To halve the width of the confidence interval, the researcher would have to

a. weigh approximately 50 people instead of 101.
b. weigh approximately 202 people instead of 101.
c. weigh approximately 303 people instead of 101.
d. weigh approximately 404 people instead of 101.
e. weigh the men in his original sample more precisely than he did.

7. By halving the width of the confidence interval, what effect is produced on the researcher's estimate of the population mean?

a. Precision is halved.
b. Precision is doubled.
c. Precision is quadrupled.
d. Bias is reduced.
e. Bias is increased.

8. Assume that the researcher had opted to weigh a random sample of adult males (n = 101) jogging in Central Park, and that he found that their mean weight was 65 kg, with a standard deviation of 9. He calculates the estimated standard error and determines the 95% confidence interval of his estimate of the population mean. Compared to the estimate obtained in the original study above (Question 3), this new estimate will be

a. less precise and less accurate.
b. less precise and equally accurate.
c. more precise and more accurate.
d. less precise and more accurate.
e. more precise and less accurate.

Question 9

One hundred oncologists were asked to estimate the mean survival time of patients with a certain type of tumor. There was very little random variation among their estimates, but their estimates proved to be consistently very pessimistic. A study of actual patients with this disease revealed that they lived, on average, 4 months longer than the oncologists estimated. Their estimate was

a. imprecise.
b. unbiased.
c. precise and biased.
d. imprecise and unbiased.
e. precise and unbiased.

3

Hypothesis Testing

Chapter 2 showed how a statistic (such as the mean of a sample) can be used to estimate a parameter (such as the mean of a population) with a known degree of confidence. This is an important use of inferential statistics, but a more important use is *hypothesis testing*.

Hypothesis testing may seem complex at first, but the steps involved are actually very simple and will be explained in this chapter. To test a hypothesis about a mean, the steps are as follows:

1. State the null and alternative hypotheses, H_O and H_A.

2. Select the decision criterion α (or "level of significance").

3. Establish the critical values.

4. Draw a random sample from the population, and calculate the mean of that sample.

5. Calculate the standard deviation (S) and estimated standard error of the sample ($s_{\bar{x}}$).

6. Calculate the value of the test statistic t that corresponds to the mean of the sample (t_{calc}).

7. Compare the calculated value of t with the critical values of t, and then accept or reject the null hypothesis.

STEP 1: STATE THE NULL AND ALTERNATIVE HYPOTHESES

Consider the following example. The dean of a medical school states that the school's students are a highly intelligent group with an average IQ of 135. This claim is a hypothesis that can be tested; it is called the **null hypothesis,** or H_O. It has this name because in most research it is the hypothesis for which there is no difference between samples or populations being compared (e.g., that a new drug produces no change compared with a placebo). If this hypothesis is rejected as false, then there is an **alternative hypothesis, H_A,** which logically must be accepted. In the case of the school president's claim, the following hypotheses can be stated:

$$\text{Null hypothesis, } H_O: \mu = 135$$

$$\text{Alternative hypothesis, } H_A: \mu \neq 135$$

One way of testing the null hypothesis would be to measure the IQ of every student in the school—in other words, to test the entire population—but this would be expensive and time-consuming. It would be more practical to draw a random sample of students, find their mean IQ, and then draw an inference from this sample.

STEP 2: SELECT THE DECISION CRITERION α

If the null hypothesis were correct, would the mean IQ of the sample of students be expected to be exactly 135? No, of course not. As shown in Chapter 2, sampling error will always cause the mean of the sample to deviate from the mean of the population. For example, if the mean IQ of the sample were 134, one might reasonably conclude that the null hypothesis was not contradicted, because sampling error could easily permit a sample with this mean to have been drawn from a population with a mean of 135. To reach a conclusion about the null hypothesis, it must therefore be decided *at what point is the difference between the sample mean and 135 not due to chance* but due to the fact that the population mean is *not* really 135, as the null hypothesis claims?

This point must be set before the sample is drawn and the data are collected. Instead of setting it in terms of the actual IQ score, it is set in terms of probability. The probability level at which it is decided that the null hypothesis is incorrect constitutes a **criterion,** or significance level, known as α (alpha).

As the random sampling distribution of means (Fig. 2–2) showed, it is unlikely that a random sample mean will be *very* different from the true population mean. If it is very different, lying far toward one of the tails of the curve, it arouses suspicion that the sample was *not* drawn from the population specified in the null hypothesis, but from a different population. [If a coin is tossed repeatedly and 5, 10, or 20 heads occur in a row, one would start to question the unstated assumption, or null hypothesis, that it was a fair coin (i.e., H_o: heads = tails in the population)]. In other words, the greater the difference between the sample mean and the population mean specified by the null hypothesis, the less probable it is that the sample really does come from the specified population. When this probability is very low, it can be concluded that the null hypothesis is incorrect.

How low does this probability need to be for the null hypothesis to be rejected as incorrect? By convention, the null hypothesis will be rejected if the probability that the sample mean could have come from the hypothesized population is less than or equal to .05; thus, the conventional level of α is .05. Conversely, if the probability of obtaining the sample mean is greater than .05, the null hypothesis will be accepted as correct. Although α may be set lower than the conventional .05 (for reasons which will be shown later), it is not normally any higher than this.

STEP 3: ESTABLISH THE CRITICAL VALUES

In Chapter 2 it was shown that if a very large number of random samples are taken from any population, their means form a normal distribution—the random sampling distribution of means—which has a mean ($\mu_{\bar{x}}$) equal to the population mean (μ). It was also shown that one can state what random sample means are so high or so low that they would occur in only 5% or fewer of all possible random samples. This ability can now be put to use, because the problem of testing the null hypothesis about the students' mean IQ involves stating which random sample means are so high or so low that they would occur in only 5% (or fewer) of all random samples that could be drawn from a population with a mean of 135.

If the sample mean falls inside the range within which 95% of random sample means would be expected to fall, the null hypothesis is accepted. This range is therefore called the **area of acceptance.** If the sample mean falls outside this range, in the **area of rejection,** the null hypothesis is rejected, and the alternative hypothesis is accepted.

The limits of this range are called the **critical values,** and they are established by referring to a table of t scores.

In the current example, the following values can be calculated:

- The sample size is 10, so there are $(n - 1) = 9$ degrees of freedom.

- The table of t scores (Table 2–1) shows that when $df = 9$, the value of t that divides the 95% (.95) area of acceptance from the two 2.5% (.025) areas of rejection is ± 2.262. These are the critical values, which are written $t_{crit} = \pm 2.262$.

Figure 3–1 shows the random sampling distribution of means for our hypothesized population with a mean (μ) of 135. It also shows the areas of rejection and acceptance defined by the critical values of t that were just established. As shown, the hypothesized population mean is sometimes written μ_{hyp}.

The following have now been established:

- the null and alternative hypotheses

- the criterion that will determine when the null hypothesis will be accepted or rejected

- the critical values of t associated with this criterion

A random sample of students can now be drawn from the population; the t score (t_{calc}) associated with their mean IQ can then be calculated and compared with the critical values of t. This is a t-test—a very common test in medical literature.

STEP 4: DRAW A RANDOM SAMPLE FROM THE POPULATION AND CALCULATE THE MEAN OF THAT SAMPLE

A random sample of 10 students is drawn; their IQs are as follows:

$$115 \ldots 140 \ldots 133 \ldots 125 \ldots 120 \ldots 126 \ldots 136 \ldots 124 \ldots 132 \ldots 129$$

The mean ($\overline{X}$) of this sample is 128.

STEP 5: CALCULATE THE STANDARD DEVIATION (*S*) AND ESTIMATED STANDARD ERROR OF THE SAMPLE ($s_{\overline{x}}$)

To calculate the t score corresponding to the sample mean, the estimated standard error must first be found. This is done as described in Chapter 2. The standard deviation (S) of this sample is calculated and found to be 7.155. The estimated standard error ($s_{\overline{x}}$) is then calculated as follows:

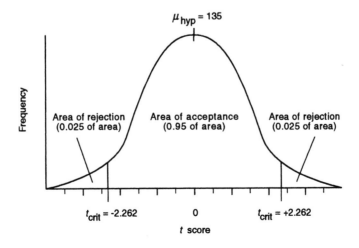

Figure 3-1

$$s_{\bar{x}} = \frac{S}{\sqrt{n-1}}$$

$$= \frac{7.155}{\sqrt{10-1}}$$

$$= 2.385$$

STEP 6: CALCULATE THE VALUE OF t THAT CORRESPONDS TO THE MEAN OF THE SAMPLE (t_{CALC})

Now that the estimated standard error has been determined, the t score corresponding to the sample mean can be found. It is the number of estimated standard errors by which the sample mean lies above or below the hypothesized population mean:

$$t = \frac{\bar{X} - \mu_{hyp}}{s_{\bar{x}}}$$

$$= \frac{128 - 135}{2.385}$$

$$= -2.935$$

So the sample mean (129) lies approximately 2.9 estimated standard errors below the hypothesized population mean (135).

STEP 7: COMPARE THE CALCULATED VALUE OF t WITH THE CRITICAL VALUES OF t, AND THEN ACCEPT OR REJECT THE NULL HYPOTHESIS

If the calculated value of t associated with the sample mean falls at or beyond either of the critical values, it is within one of the two areas of rejection.

Figure 3–2 shows that the t score in this example **does** fall within the lower area of rejection. Therefore, the null hypothesis is rejected, and alternative hypothesis is accepted.

The reasoning behind this is as follows. The sample mean differs so much from the hypothesized population mean that the probability that it would have been obtained if the null hypothesis were true is only .05 (or less). Because this probability is so low, it is concluded that the population mean is not 135. It can be said that the difference between the sample mean and the hypothesized population mean is **statistically significant,** and that the null hypothesis has been rejected at the .05 level. This would typically be reported as follows: "The hypothesis that the mean IQ of the population is 135 was rejected, $t = -2.935$, $df = 9$, $p \leq .05$."

If, on the other hand, the calculated value of t associated with the sample mean fell between the two critical values, in the area of acceptance, the null hypothesis would be accepted instead. In such a case, it would be said that the difference between the sample mean and the hypothesized population mean failed to reach statistical significance ($p > .05$).

Z-TESTS

References to a "z-test" are sometimes made in medical literature. A z-test involves the same steps as a t-test and can be used when the sample is large enough ($n > 100$) for the sample standard deviation to provide a reliable estimate of the standard error. Although there are situations in which a t-test can be used but a z-test cannot, there are no situations in which a z-test can be used but a t-test cannot. Therefore, t-tests are the more important and widely used of the two.

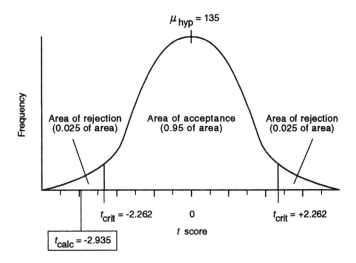

Figure 3-2

THE MEANING OF STATISTICAL SIGNIFICANCE

When a result is reported to be "significant at $p \leq .05$," it merely means *that the result was unlikely to have occurred by chance*—in this case, that the likelihood of the result having occurred by chance is .05 or less. This does *not* necessarily mean that the result is truly "significant" in the everyday meaning of the word—that it is important, note-worthy, or meaningful. Nor does it mean that it is necessarily clinically significant.

In the previous example, if the mean IQ of the sample of students was found to be 134, it is possible (if the sample were large enough) that this mean could fall in the area of rejection, and so the null hypothesis ($\mu = 135$) could be rejected. However, this would scarcely be an important or noteworthy disproof of the dean's claim about the students' intelligence. (In fact, virtually *any* null hypothesis can be rejected if the sample is sufficiently large, because there will almost always be some trivial difference between the hypothesized mean and the sample mean. Studies using extremely large samples are therefore at risk of producing findings that are statistically significant but otherwise insignificant).

Similarly, a study of a diet drug versus a placebo might conclude that the drug was effective. Nevertheless, if the difference in weight was only 1 pound, this would not be a significant finding in the usual meaning of the word, and would probably not lead to physicians prescribing the drug.

TYPE I AND TYPE II ERRORS

A statement that a result is "significant at $p \leq .05$" means that an investigator can be 95% sure that the result was not obtained by chance. It also means that there is a 5% probability that the result *could* have been obtained by chance. Although the null hypothesis is being rejected, it *could* still be true: there remains a 5% chance that the data *did*, in fact, come from the population specified by the null hypothesis.[1]

Questions on types I and II errors will appear not only on Step 1, but also on Step 2, Step 3, and even specialty board certification examinations.

Rejecting the null hypothesis when it is true is a **type I** or **"false-negative" error:** a false-negative conclusion has been drawn about the null hypothesis. The probability that a type I error is being made is in fact the value of *p;* because this value relates to the criterion α, a type I error is also known as an **alpha error.**

 The opposite kind of error, accepting the null hypothesis when it is actually false (drawing a **"false-positive"** conclusion) is a **type II** or **beta error.** Whereas the probability of making a type I error is α, the probability of making a type II error is β. Table 3–1 shows the four possible types of decisions that can be made on the basis of statistical tests.

The choice of an appropriate level for the criterion α therefore depends on the relative consequences of making a type I or type II error. For example, if a study is expensive and time-consuming (and is therefore unlikely to be repeated), yet has important practical implications, the researchers may wish to establish a more stringent level of α (such as .01, .005, or even .001) to be more than 95% sure that their conclusions are correct. This was done in the multimillion dollar Lipid Research Clinics Coronary Primary Prevention Trial, whose planners stated that

> since the time, magnitude, and costs of this study make it unlikely that it could ever be repeated, it was essential that any observed benefit of total cholesterol lowering was a real one. Therefore, α was set to .01 rather than the usual .05. (Lipid Research Clinics Program, 1979)

Although the criterion to be selected need not be .05, by convention it cannot be any higher. Results that do not quite reach the .05 level of probability are sometimes reported to "approach significance" or to "show statistically significant trends."

Many researchers do not state a predetermined criterion or report their results in terms of one; instead, they report the actual probability that the obtained result could have occurred by chance if the null hypothesis were true (e.g., "*p* = .015"). In these cases, the *p* value is more an "index of rarity" than a true decision criterion. The researchers are showing how unlikely it is that a type I error has been made, even though they would have still rejected the null hypothesis if the outcome were only significant at the .05 level.

POWER OF STATISTICAL TESTS

Although it is possible to guard against a type I error simply by using a more stringent (lower) level of α, preventing a type II error is not so easy. Because a type II error involves accepting a false null hypothesis, the ability of a statistical test to avoid a type II error depends on its ability to detect a null hypothesis that is false. This ability is called the **power** of the test, and it is equal to 1 − β: it is the probability that a false null hypothesis will be rejected. Conventionally, a study is required to have a power of 0.8 to be acceptable—in other words, a study that has a less than 80% chance of detecting a false null hypothesis is generally judged to be unacceptable.

Calculating β and determining the power of a test is complex. Nevertheless, it is clear that a test's power, or ability to detect a false null hypothesis, will increase as:

- α increases (e.g., from .01 to .05). This will make the critical values of *t* less extreme, thus increasing the size of the areas of rejection and making rejection of the null hypothesis more likely. There will always be a trade-off between type I and type II errors: increasing α reduces the chance of a type II error, but it simultaneously increases the chance of a type I error.

- the size of the difference between the sample mean and the hypothesized population mean increases (this is known as the effect size). In the preceding example, a difference between a hypothesized population mean IQ of 135 and a sample mean IQ of 100 would be detected much more easily (and hence the null hypothesis would be rejected more easily) than a difference between a hypothesized IQ of 135

Table 3-1

		ACTUAL SITUATION	
		H_o True	H_o False
	H_o Accepted	Correct	Type II error (β) False positive
	H_o Rejected	Type I error (α) False negative	Correct

(Row labels at left, reading vertically: **T E S T   R E S U L T**)

and a sample mean IQ of 128. The larger the difference, the more extreme the calculated value of t.

- sampling error decreases. A lower sampling error means that the sample standard deviation (S) is reduced, which will cause the estimated standard error ($s_{\bar{x}}$) to be lower. Because t is calculated in terms of estimated standard errors, this will make the calculated value of t more extreme (whether in a positive or negative direction), increasing the likelihood that it falls in one of the areas of rejection.

- the sample size (n) increases; this reduces the estimated standard error ($s_{\bar{x}}$), thereby increasing the calculated value of t. Therefore, a large-scale study is more likely to detect a false null hypothesis (particularly if the effect-size is small) than is a small-scale study. For example, if a coin is tossed 1000 times and results in 600 heads and 400 tails, one is much more able to reject the null hypothesis that the coin is a fair one than if the coin is tossed 10 times and 6 heads and 4 tails are obtained.

 Increasing the sample size is the most practical and important way of increasing the power of a statistical test.

Researchers who dispute the findings of a study in which the null hypothesis is accepted, claiming that it is an example of a type II error, may argue that the study's sample was too small to detect a real difference or effect. They may replicate the study using a larger sample to improve the likelihood of getting statistically significant results that will allow them to reject the null hypothesis.

In practice, researchers try to predict the effect size before they begin a study, so that they can use a sample size large enough to detect it. They do not simply guess, for instance, that 50 or 500 patients will be needed to test a new drug. Ideally, all studies that report acceptance of the null hypothesis should also report the power of the test used, so that the risk of a type II error is made clear.

The concept of power can be explained by using the example of a military radar system that is being used to detect a possible impending air attack. The null hypothesis is that there are no aircraft or missiles approaching; the alternative hypothesis is that there are. Clearly, a powerful radar system is going to be more able to detect intruders than is a weak one.

What if the radar system is functioning at a very lower power, and the operators are not aware of this fact? They watch their screens and report that the null hypothesis is correct—there are no aircraft or missiles approaching—but the power of their system is so low that they are in great danger of making a type II, or false-positive, error. This danger is greater if the "effect size"—the difference between the presence or absence of impending attackers—is likely to be low: a lone saboteur in a hang-glider will only be detected by a very powerful system, while a low-powered system may be adequate to detect a squadron of large bombers. So just as with a statistical test, the more subtle the phenomenon being testing for, the more powerful the test needs to be.

On the other hand, a very powerful system—like a very powerful statistical test—runs the risk of making a type I error. A phenomenon so subtle as to be trivial, such as a flock of birds, may produce a signal, which may lead the operators to reject the null hypothesis and conclude that an attack is on the way.

DIRECTIONAL HYPOTHESES

So far, the example of hypothesis testing has used a **nondirectional** alternative hypothesis, which merely stated that the population mean is *not* equal to 135, but it did not specify whether the population mean is above or below this figure. This was appropriate because the medical school dean claimed that the students' mean IQ was 135. His claim (which constitutes the null hypothesis) could legitimately be rejected if the sample mean IQ turned out to be significantly above *or* below 135. Therefore, as Figure 3–2 showed, there were *two* areas of rejection, one above μ_{hyp} and one below.

What if the dean had instead claimed that the students' average IQ was at *least* 135? This claim could only be rejected if the sample mean IQ turned out to be significantly *lower* than 135. The null hypothesis is now $\mu \geq 135$, and the alternative hypothesis must now be $\mu < 135$. The alternative hypothesis is now a **directional** one, which specifies that the population mean lies in a *particular direction* with respect to the null hypothesis.

In this kind of situation, there are no longer two areas of rejection on the random sampling distribution of means. As Figure 3–3 shows, there is now only one. If α remains at .05, the area of acceptance (the area in which 95% of the means of possible samples drawn from the hypothesized population lie) now extends down from the very top end of the distribution, leaving just *one* area of rejection—the bottom 5% of the curve. The area of rejection now lies in only one tail of the distribution, rather than in both tails.

The steps involved in conducting a *t*-test of this directional null hypothesis are exactly the same as before, except that the critical value of *t* is now different. The critical value now divides the bottom 5% tail of the distribution from the upper 95%, instead of dividing the middle 95% from two tails of 2.5% each. The appropriate column of Table 2–1 shows that the new critical value of *t* (for the same *df* of 9) is −1.833, rather than the previous value of ±2.262.

As Figure 3–3 shows, this new critical value is associated with only one tail of the distribution. Using this value therefore involves performing a **one-tailed** statistical test, due to the fact that the alternative hypothesis is directional; previously, when the alternative hypothesis was nondirectional, the test performed was a **two-tailed** test.

The critical value of *t* is less extreme for the one-tailed test (−1.833) than for the two-tailed test (±2.262). Consequently, when a one-tailed test is used, a less extreme sample mean is able to exceed the critical value and fall within the area of rejection, leading to rejection of the null hypothesis. As a result of this, **one-tailed tests are more powerful than two-tailed tests.**

For example, if the mean IQ of the sample of 10 students were 130 (instead of 128), with the same standard deviation (7.155) and the same estimated standard error (2.385) as before, the value of *t* corresponding to this mean would be

$$\frac{130 - 135}{2.385} = -2.096$$

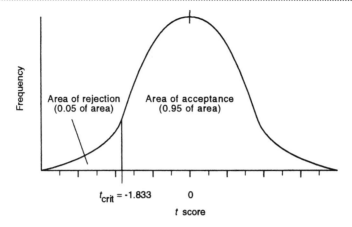

Figure 3-3

This score falls within the area of acceptance for a two-tailed test, but it falls within the area of rejection for a one-tailed test, as shown in Figure 3–3. The dean's claim could therefore potentially be accepted *or* rejected, depending on how it is interpreted and which test is consequently performed.

As this example shows, a researcher who wishes to reject the null hypothesis may sometimes find that using a one-tailed rather than a two-tailed test allows a previously nonsignificant result to become significant. For this reason it is important that one-tailed tests are only performed under the correct conditions. The decision to use a one-tailed test must depend on *the nature of the hypothesis being tested, and should therefore be decided at the outset of the research*, rather than being decided afterward according to how the results turn out.

One-tailed tests can only be used when there is a directional alternative hypothesis. This means that they may not be used unless results in only one direction are of interest, and the possibility of the results being in the opposite direction is of no interest or consequence to the researcher.

When testing a new drug, the normal null hypothesis is that the drug has no effect, so it will be rejected if the drug turns out to have an effect too great to be due to chance, irrespective of whether the effect is a positive one or a negative one. Although the researcher *expects* the drug to produce an improvement in patients' symptoms, this expectation does not permit the use of a directional alternative hypothesis. The researcher can do this only if it is of no interest or consequence if the drug actually makes patients worse—a claim that can almost never be made legitimately in biomedical research.

TESTING FOR DIFFERENCES BETWEEN GROUPS

We have seen how a *t*-test can be used to test a hypothesis about a single mean. However, biomedical research is often more complex than this: researchers commonly want to compare *two* means, such as the effects of two different drugs or the mean survival times of patients receiving two different treatments.

A slightly more complex version of the *t*-test can be used to test for a significant difference between two means. The null hypothesis is that the two groups were drawn from populations with the same mean—in other words, that the two samples were in effect drawn from the same population, and that there is no difference between them. The alternative hypothesis is that the two population means are different:

$$H_O : \mu_A = \mu_B$$
$$H_A : \mu_A \neq \mu_B$$

Many research problems involve comparing *more than two groups*; for example, comparing the treatment outcomes of three groups of patients with depression—one group taking a placebo, another a tricyclic antidepressant, the third a selective serotonin reuptake inhibitor (SSRI). If each group consists of male and female patients, the researcher may also want to make comparisons between the sexes, giving a total of six groups: three different treatment groups, with two sexes within each group. Therefore, the null hypothesis is

$$H_O : \mu_A = \mu_B = \mu_C = \mu_D = \mu_E = \mu_F$$

In theory, this hypothesis could be tested by multiple *t*-tests, comparing A with B, A with C, A with D, A with E, A with F, B with C, and so on. However, this method has some important disadvantages:

- It is time-consuming because it involves performing 15 separate *t*-tests.

- The power of each test is relatively low because each test uses the elements in only two groups, and not the sample as a whole.

- With an α of .05, each test has a .05 chance of producing a type I error; with 15 tests, the probability of at least one of them producing a type I error is unacceptably high.

- The 15 tests will produce 15 separate specific answers (e.g., "men taking an SSRI responded better than women taking a placebo").

It would be more convenient if an *overall* answer were first obtained to see if there were *any* statistically significant differences in the data. Then, broad questions such as, "Is there a significant difference between the three treatments?" could be answered before finally looking for significant differences between subgroups. This is especially true if the researcher has some general expectations (e.g., that men with depression have a better prognosis than women with depression) but has no specific expectations about differences between particular subgroups.

Fortunately, there is a technique that overcomes these problems: **analysis of variance** (or **ANOVA**). Whereas a *t*-test is appropriate for making just one comparison (between two sample means, or between a sample mean and a hypothesized population mean), when more than one comparison is being made (i.e., when means of more than two groups are being compared), ANOVA is the appropriate technique. Consequently, ANOVA is used very commonly.

ANALYSIS OF VARIANCE (ANOVA)

The actual computation of ANOVA is complex and is not required for the USMLE. Briefly, the logic behind it is as follows. In any set of experimental results, such as the results of the study of antidepressant drugs in the previous section, there will be some variability. The total variability in the results is made up of two components:

1. The variability resulting from the known differences between the groups: the use of the placebo, the tricyclic antidepressant, or the SSRI as well as the gender of the patient.

2. The ordinary random variability within each group that is to be expected in any set of data, caused by sampling error, individual differences between the patients, and so on.

The essential question is this: can a significant proportion of the overall variability found in the results be attributed to the known differences between the groups or not? If the variance between the different groups is large in comparison with the random fluctuations found within the groups, then it must be due to some difference between the groups above and beyond the random fluctuations. If the experiment has been performed correctly, this difference must be due (in this example) to the gender of the patients or the treatments that they were given, because there is no other nonrandom difference between the groups.

The F-ratio

ANOVA compares variance by means of a simple ratio, which is called the **F-ratio:**

$$F = \frac{\text{variance between groups}}{\text{variance within groups}}$$

The resulting F statistic (F_{calc}) is then compared with the critical value of F (F_{crit}), obtained from F tables in much the same way as was done with t. As with t, if the calculated value exceeds the critical value for the appropriate level of α, the null hypothesis will be rejected. An **F-test** is therefore a test of the *ratio of variances*.

F-tests can also be used on their own, independently of the ANOVA technique, to test hypotheses about variances. For example, two different vaccines (A and B) may produce the same mean antibody concentration, but one vaccine may produce levels that are more variable than the other. An F-test would be used to establish if the difference in their variances is merely due to chance or is statistically significant. The null hypothesis would be $\sigma^2_A = \sigma^2_B$.

In ANOVA, the F-test is used to establish whether a statistically significant difference exists in the data being tested. It will show if there are significant sources of variability in the data above and beyond the expected random variability.

If the various experimental groups differ in terms of only one factor at a time—such as the type of drug being used—a **one-way** ANOVA is used. If the variance between groups is sufficiently large, compared with the variance within groups, for the F-ratio to reach significance, it would then be known that drug type was a significant source of variation in the results.

On the other hand, if the various groups differ in terms of two factors at a time, then a **two-way** ANOVA is performed. This is what would be required if the groups differ not only in terms of drug type but also in terms of gender. This ANOVA will show not only if there are significant sources of variability in the results—it will also show if this variability is attributable to one factor (drug type), to the other factor (gender), or to the two factors in combination with each other.

If a single factor is found to have a significant effect, it is called a **main effect.** If a combination of factors has a significant effect, this is called an **interaction effect.** Interaction effects occur when the effect of two factors together differs from the sum of the individual effects of each alone.

Graphical presentations of ANOVA data

Main and interaction effects are more easily understood visually. In the example of the study of the effects of SSRIs, tricyclics, and placebos on male and female patients with depression, assume that the results show that the best outcomes were among the patients who took the tricyclics, followed by those who took the SSRIs, and that the worst outcomes were among the patients who took the placebo; also assume that there are no differences attributable to the gender of the patients.

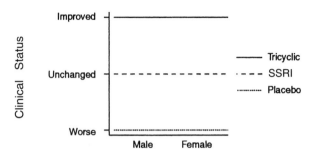

Figure 3-4

Figure 3–4 shows these results. Provided the differences are large enough to reach statistical significance, a two-way ANOVA would allow the conclusion that there is a main effect due to drug type, that there is no effect due to patient gender, and that there is no effect due to an interaction between drug type and patient gender.

Now assume that in addition to these drug effects, female patients had better outcomes than male patients in each of the three treatment groups. Figure 3–5 illustrates this result; here there is a main effect of drug, a main effect of gender, and no interaction effect.

Now assume instead that the three different treatments all produced identical results, and yet the female patients still exhibited better outcomes within each of these treatment groups. Figure 3–6 shows this result; here there is a main effect of gender but no main effect of drug and no interaction effect.

Figure 3–7 shows another possible result. The three treatment groups produce identical *mean* effects when both sexes are considered together; the male and female patient groups have identical *mean* outcomes when all three drugs are considered together; but there are strong effects associated with particular *combinations* of gender and drug type.

In this situation, although there is no main effect of drug and no main effect of gender, there is, nevertheless, a strong *interaction effect* of drug and gender (this would usually be reported as "a strong drug × gender interaction"). Overall, the drugs have no effect, and gender has no effect, but there are strong effects of particular combinations of drug and gender.

When the lines representing different groups on graphs of this kind are parallel, there are no inter-

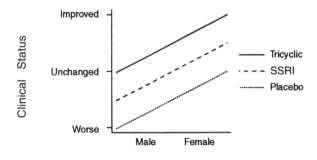

Figure 3-5

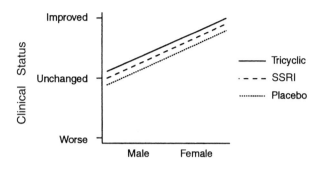

Figure 3-6

actions. When they are not parallel, an interaction effect is present (although it is not necessarily a strong or statistically significant one). Interaction effects reach maximum strength when the lines are at right angles to each other.

An example helps to understand the difference between main effects and interaction effects. Ask yourself the following questions:

• Is it socially stigmatizing to wear a beard in public?

• Is it socially stigmatizing to wear lipstick in public?

The answer, in most cultures, is "It depends"—on whether we are talking about men or women. Whenever the answer is "It depends," an interaction effect is likely to be present. We cannot say whether it is stigmatizing to wear a beard or lipstick in general—in other words, there is no main effect of beard- or lipstick-wearing on social stigmatization—but there clearly is an interaction between type of facial adornment and gender on social stigmatization. Men who wear lipstick and women who wear beards are at risk of being stigmatized, even though there is nothing "wrong" with either lipstick or beards *in general*. Again, when represented graphically (Figure 3–8), note that the lines are at right angles to each other, signifying a strong interaction.

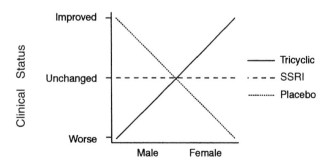

Figure 3-7

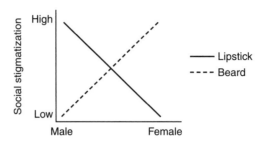

Figure 3-8

NONPARAMETRIC AND DISTRIBUTION-FREE TESTS

The previous sections have dealt with t-, z-, and F-tests, which test hypotheses about means or variances. These tests share three common features:

- Their hypotheses refer to *population parameters*: the population mean (in the case of t- and z-tests) or the population variance (in the case of F-tests). For this reason such tests are called **parametric** tests.

- Their hypotheses concern *interval* or *ratio* scale data, such as weight, blood pressure, IQ, per capita income, measures of clinical improvement, and so on.

- They make certain assumptions about the distribution of the data of interest in the population—principally, that the population data are normally distributed. (As was shown earlier, the central limit theorem allows this assumption to be made, even when little is known about the population distribution, provided that random samples of sufficient size are used).

There are other statistical techniques that do not share these features:

- They do not test hypotheses concerning parameters, and hence are known as **nonparametric tests.**

- They do not assume that the population is normally distributed, so they are also called **distribution-free tests.**

- They are used to test nominal or ordinal scale data.

Such tests, however, have the disadvantage that they are generally *less powerful* than parametric tests.

Chi-square

The most important nonparametric test is the **chi-square** (χ^2) test, which is used for testing hypotheses about *nominal scale* data.

Chi-square is basically a test of *proportions*, telling us whether the proportions of observations falling in different categories differ significantly from the proportions that would be expected by chance.

For example, in tossing a coin 100 times, we would expect 50% (or 50) of the tosses to fall in the category of heads and 50 to fall in the category of tails. If the result is 59 heads and 41 tails,

Table 3-2

Number of Students Passing USMLE by Medical School			
	School A	School B	School C
Number Passing	49	112	26	Total 187
Number Failing	12	37	8	Total 57
Total	61	149	34	

chi-square would show whether this difference in proportion is too large to be expected by chance (i.e., whether it is statistically significant).

As with other tests, chi-square involves calculating the test statistic (χ^2_{calc}) according to a standard formula and comparing it with the critical value (appropriate for the level of α selected) shown in the published chi-square tables. These tables can be found in most statistics textbooks.

Chi-square is also used in more complicated nominal scale questions. For example, a study might compare the USMLE pass rates of three different medical schools, as shown in Table 3–2. This kind of table is a **contingency table,** which is the usual way of presenting this kind of data. It expresses the idea that one variable (such as passing or failing the examination) may be contingent on the other (such as which medical school one attended). The question that chi-square can answer is this: is there a relationship between which school the student attended and passing or failing the examination?

NOTE

[1]Many statistics textbooks and researchers erroneously take this to mean that there is therefore a 5% chance that the null hypothesis is in fact still true, although it is being rejected. The *p* or α value is the probability that the data could have come from the population specified by the null hypothesis, *not* the other way around (Hill, 1990).

EXERCISES

Select the single, best answer to the following questions.

1. An investigation of the effectiveness of a new drug using chi-square reports $\chi^2 = 4.6$, p $\leq$ .05. This means that

a. if the drug were effective, the probability of this result is .05.
b. the researchers are 95% certain that the drug is ineffective.
c. if the drug were ineffective, the probability of this result is .05.
d. the study was not powerful enough to detect a real effect of the drug.
e. the result is not statistically significant

2. A study rejects the null hypothesis that the mean duration of viral shedding in primary HSV-1 infections is 7 days, $t = 2.935$, $df = 9$, $p < .05$. This means that

a. 5% of the cases did have a mean duration of viral shedding of 7 days.
b. the mean duration of viral shedding was 9 days.
c. there is a 5% chance that a case would have less than 7 days of viral shedding.
d. there is a 5% chance that the null hypothesis is being rejected incorrectly.
e. the sample size was only 10, which is unlikely to be large enough to allow a statistically significant result to be obtained.

3. A chi-square test would be most appropriate for testing which one of the following hypotheses?

a. That the mean USMLE Step 1 score of Harvard students is greater than that of Stanford students.
b. That a smaller proportion of people who were immunized against chicken pox subsequently develop zoster than those who were not immunized.
c. That the mean blood pressure of black and white male hypertensive patients taking ACE inhibitors is the same as that of black and white female hypertensive patients taking ACE inhibitors and that of black and white males and females taking diuretics and placebos.
d. That race interacts with the type of drug used to treat hypertension.
e. That the mean cost of treating a patient with coronary artery disease with angioplasty is greater than the mean cost of providing medical treatment.

4. An analysis of variance (ANOVA) technique would be the most appropriate technique for testing which one of the following hypotheses?

a. That the mean indebtedness on graduation is greater for students at private rather than public medical schools.
b. That a smaller proportion of vegetarians rather than nonvegetarians develop colon cancer by age 70.
c. That the mean blood pressure of black and white male hypertensive patients taking ACE inhibitors is that same as that of black and white female hypertensive patients taking ACE inhibitors and that of black and white males and females taking diuretics and placebos.
d. That a larger proportion of black people than white people treated for hypertension with ACE inhibitors suffer strokes.
e. That the mean length of hospital stay for patients admitted with pneumonia is greater under fee-for-service insurance plans than capitated plans.

Questions 5–7

A medical student believes that interns get less sleep than the general population of young adults. He decides to test this hypothesis by taking a random sample of 10 interns on 2 randomly selected days, and asking them how many hours they slept the previous night. He then compares their mean number of hours of sleep with that of the general population of young adults, which he assumes to be 8 hours per night. He selects an alpha of .05.

5. All the following statements are true EXCEPT

a. H_0: interns' mean sleep duration $= 8$; H_A: interns' mean sleep duration $\neq 8$.
b. Because there is no real reason to suppose that interns' hours of sleep are normally distributed, a t-test would be inappropriate.

c. The 95% confidence limits for his estimate of the true number of hours slept by interns is the sample mean plus or minus approximately 2 times the estimated sample error.
d. A two-tailed test should be used.
e. The student has a 5% chance of making a type I error.

6. If he selected an alpha of 0.01, he would

a. be more likely to obtain a statistically significant result.
b. be less likely to make a type II error.
c. be more likely to make a type I error.
d. be more confident of his findings if they were statistically significant.
e. have a more powerful study.

7. If his findings were not statistically significant, this result could be due to all of the following EXCEPT

a. The sample size was too large.
b. The null hypothesis really was true.
c. The size of the difference between the interns' number of hours sleep and 8 was too small to be detected.
d. The study was lacking in power.

4

Correlational Techniques

Biomedical research often seeks to establish if there is a relationship between two variables; for example, is there a relationship between salt intake and blood pressure, or between cigarette smoking and life expectancy? The methods used to do this are **correlational** techniques, which focus on the "co-relatedness" of the two variables. There are two basic kinds of correlational techniques:

- **Correlation,** which is used to establish and quantify the *strength* and *direction* of the relationship between two variables.

- **Regression,** which is used to express the *functional relationship* between two variables, so that the value of one variable can be *predicted* from knowledge of the other.

CORRELATION

Correlation simply expresses the strength and direction of the relationship between two variables in terms of a **correlation coefficient,** signified by r. Values of r vary from -1 to $+1$; the strength of the relationship is indicated by the size of the coefficient, while its direction is indicated by the sign.

A plus sign means that there is a **positive correlation** between the two variables—high values of one variable (such as salt intake) are associated with high values of the other variable (such as blood pressure). A minus sign means that there is a **negative correlation** between the two variables—high values of one variable (such as cigarette consumption) are associated with low values of the other (such as life expectancy).

If there is a "perfect" linear relationship between the two variables, so that it is possible to know the exact value of one variable from knowledge of the other variable, the correlation coefficient (r) will be exactly plus or minus 1.00. If there is absolutely no relationship between the two variables, so that it is impossible to know anything about one variable on the basis of knowledge of the other variable, then the coefficient will be zero. Coefficients beyond ± 0.5 are typically regarded as strong, whereas coefficients between zero and ± 0.5 are usually regarded as weak.

Scattergrams and bivariate distributions

The relationship between two correlated variables forms a **bivariate distribution,** which is commonly presented graphically in the form of a **scattergram.** The first variable (salt intake, cigarette consumption) is usually plotted on the horizontal (X) axis, and the second variable (blood pressure, life expectancy) is plotted on the vertical (Y) axis. Each plotted data point represents one observation of a pair of values, such as one patient's salt intake and blood pressure, so the number of plotted points is equal to the sample size n. Figure 4–1 shows four different scattergrams.

Determining a correlation coefficient involves mathematically finding the "line of best fit" to the plotted data points. The relationship between the appearance of the scattergram and the correlation

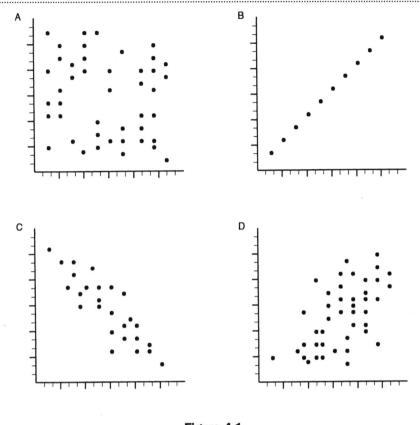

Figure 4-1

coefficient can therefore be understood by imagining how well a straight line could fit the plotted points. In Figure 4–1A, for example, it is not possible to draw any straight line that would fit the plotted points *at all*; therefore, the correlation coefficient is approximately zero. In Figure 4–1B, a straight line would fit the plotted points perfectly—so the correlation coefficient is 1.00. Figure 4–1C shows a strong negative correlation, with a correlation coefficient in the region of −0.8, and Figure 4–1D shows a weak positive correlation in the region of +0.3.

Types of correlation coefficient

The two most commonly used correlation coefficients are the **Pearson product-moment correlation,** which is used for *interval* or *ratio* scale data, and the **Spearman rank-order correlation,** which is used for *ordinal* scale data. The latter is sometimes symbolized by the letter ρ (rho). Pearson's *r* would therefore be used (for example) to express the association between salt intake and blood pressure (which are both ratio scale data), whereas Spearman's ρ would be used to express the association between birth order and class position at school (which are both ordinal scale data).

Both these correlational techniques are **linear:** they evaluate the strength of a "straight line" relationship between the two variables. So if there is a very strong **nonlinear** relationship between two variables, the Pearson or Spearman correlation coefficients will be an underestimate of the true strength of the relationship.

Figure 4–2 illustrates such a situation. A drug has a strong effect at medium dosage levels but very

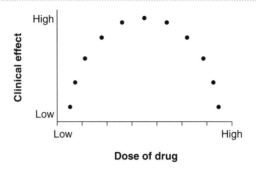

Figure 4-2   A strong nonlinear relationship.

weak effects at very high or very low doses. Because the relationship between dose and effect is so nonlinear, the Pearson r correlation coefficient is low, even though there is actually a very strong relationship between the two variables. Visual inspection of scattergrams is therefore invaluable in identifying relationships of this sort. More advanced nonlinear correlational techniques can be used to quantify correlations of this kind.

Coefficient of determination

Once a correlation coefficient has been determined, the **coefficient of determination** can be found by *squaring the value of r*. The coefficient of determination, symbolized by r^2, expresses the proportion of the variance in one variable that is accounted for, or "explained," by the variance in the other variable. So if a study finds a correlation (r) of 0.40 between salt intake and blood pressure, it could be concluded that $0.40 \times 0.40 = 0.16$, or 16% of the variance in blood pressure in this study is accounted for by variance in salt intake. This does not necessarily mean that the changes in salt intake *caused* the change in blood pressure.

 A correlation between two variables does **not** demonstrate a causal relationship between the two variables, no matter how strong it is. Correlation is merely a measure of the variables' statistical association, not of their causal relationship. *Inferring a causal relationship between two variables on the basis of a correlation is a common and fundamental error.*

Furthermore, the fact that a correlation is present between two variables in a sample does not necessarily mean that the correlation actually exists in the population. When a correlation has been found between two variables in a sample, the researcher will normally wish to test the null hypothesis that there is no correlation between the two variables (i.e., that $r = 0$) in the population. This is done with a special form of t-test.

REGRESSION

If two variables are highly correlated, it then becomes possible to *predict* the value of one of them (the dependent variable) from the value of other (the independent variable) by using **regression** techniques. In **simple linear regression** the value of one variable (X) is used to predict the value of the other variable (Y) by means of a simple linear mathematical function, the **regression equation,** which quantifies the straight-line relationship between the two variables. This straight line, or **regression line,** is actually the same "line of best fit" to the scattergram as that used in calculating the correlation coefficient.

The simple linear regression equation is the same as the equation for any straight line:

$$\text{Expected value of } Y = a + bX$$

where   a   is a constant, known as the "intercept constant" because it is the point on the Y axis where the Y axis is intercepted by the regression line;

           b   is the slope of the regression line, and is known as the **regression coefficient;** and

           X   is the value of the variable X.

Once the values of a and b have been established, the expected value of Y can be predicted for any given value of X. For example, Zito and Reid (1978) showed that the hepatic clearance rate of lidocaine (Y, in ml/min/kg) can be predicted from the hepatic clearance rate of indocyanine green dye (X, in ml/min/kg), according to the equation $Y = 0.30 + 1.07X$, thus enabling anesthesiologists to reduce the risk of lidocaine overdosage by testing clearance of the dye.

Multiple regression

Other techniques generate **multiple regression** equations, in which more than one variable is used to predict the expected value of Y, thus increasing the overall percentage of variance in Y that can be accounted for. For example, Rubin *et al.* (1986) found that the birth weight of a baby (Y, in grams) can be partly predicted from the number of cigarettes smoked on a daily basis by both the baby's mother (X_1) and the baby's father (X_2) according to the multiple regression equation $Y = 3385 - 9X_1 - 6X_2$. Other techniques are available to quantify nonlinear relationships among multiple variables. As with correlation, however, it is important to remember that the existence of this kind of statistical association is **not** in itself evidence of causality.

CHOOSING AN APPROPRIATE INFERENTIAL OR CORRELATIONAL TECHNIQUE

The basic choice of an appropriate statistical technique for a particular research problem is determined by two factors: the scale of measurement and the type of question being asked. USMLE will require familiarity with only those basic techniques that have been covered here (although there are many others). Their uses will now be summarized, as illustrated in Table 4–1.

Concerning *nominal scale data*, only one kind of question has been discussed: do the proportions of observations falling in different categories differ significantly from the proportions that would be expected by chance? The technique for such questions is the **chi-square test.**

Regarding *ordinal scale data*, only one kind of question has been mentioned: is there an association between ordinal position on one ranking and ordinal position on another ranking? The appropriate technique here is the **Spearman rank-order correlation.**

For *interval* or *ratio scale data*, three general kinds of questions have been discussed:

1. Questions concerning means:

    *   What is the true mean of the population?

    *   Is one sample mean significantly different from one or more other sample means?

2. Questions concerning variances:

    *   Are the variances in two samples significantly different?

3. Questions concerning association:

    *   To what degree are two variables correlated?

Table 4-1

		SCALE OF DATA		
		Nominal	Ordinal	Interval or Ratio
QUESTIONS CONCERNING	Differences in proportion	χ^2		
	One or two means			t-test (or z-test if $n > 100$)
	More than two means			ANOVA with F-tests
	Variances			F-test
	Association		Spearman ρ	Pearson r
	Predicting the value of a variable			Regression

Three ways of answering questions concerning *means* of interval or ratio scale data have been examined: t-tests, z-tests, and ANOVA:

- When the question involves only *one or two* means, or making only *one* comparison, a t-test will normally be used. Therefore, questions concerning estimating a population mean, testing a hypothesis about a population mean, or comparing two sample means with each other will normally be answered by using t. Alternatively, provided that $n > 100$, or if the standard deviation of the population is known, a z-test may be used with virtually identical results.

- When the question involves *more than two* means, or making *more than one* comparison, the appropriate technique is **analysis of variance** (ANOVA), together with **F-tests.**

One way of answering questions about *variances* has been covered: the **F-test** of significant differences between variances.

Two ways of assessing the *degree of association* between two interval or ratio scale variables have been discussed. To evaluate the strength and direction of the relationship, **Pearson product-moment correlation** is used, together with a form of t-test to test the null hypothesis that the relationship does not exist in the population. To make predictions about the value of one variable on the basis of the other, **regression** techniques are used.

Table 4–1 summarizes the range of inferential and correlational techniques that have been covered. This table should be memorized to answer typical USMLE questions that require choosing the correct test or technique for a given research situation.

EXERCISES

Select the single, best answer to the following questions.

1. A medical school professor finds that students' final examination grades correlate with the number of times they attended class, Pearson $r = 0.8$, $p = .001$. This means that

a. a student will improve his or her grade by attending class more.
b. 64% of the variation in final grades is accounted for by class attendance.
c. the correlation is too low to be of significance.
d. the correlation is a weak one.
e. the correlation is nonlinear.

2. A lecturer states that the correlation coefficient between prefrontal blood flow under cognitive load and the severity of psychotic symptoms in schizophrenic patients is -1.24. You can therefore conclude that

a. prefrontal blood flow under cognitive load is a good predictor of the severity of psychotic symptoms in schizophrenic patients.
b. prefrontal blood flow under cognitive load accounts for a large proportion of the variance in psychotic symptoms in schizophrenic patients.
c. low prefrontal blood flow is in some way a cause or partial cause of psychosis.
d. psychosis or schizophrenia is in some way a cause or partial cause of low prefrontal blood flow under cognitive load.
e. the lecturer has reported the correlation coefficient incorrectly.

3. An investigator into the life expectancy of IV drug abusers divides a sample of patients into HIV-positive and HIV-negative groups. What type of data does this division constitute?

a. Nominal
b. Ordinal
c. Interval
d. Ratio
e. Continuous

4. The investigator in Question 3 finds that 169 of 212 HIV-positive IV drug abusers are no longer alive after 5 years, while only 64 of 439 HIV-negative IV drug abusers have died during this time. What statistical technique should he use to test the null hypothesis that there is no difference between these proportions?

a. t-test
b. Correlation with associated t-test
c. Chi-square
d. Analysis of variance (ANOVA)
e. F-test

5. A researcher wishes to compare the effects of four different antiretroviral drug combinations on the survival time of two groups of patients with AIDS; one group are IV drug abusers, the other are infants infected *in utero*. Each of these groups is divided into four subgroups; each subgroup is given a different drug combination. Which statistical technique would be most appropriate for analyzing the results of this study?

    a. Analysis of variance (ANOVA)
    b. *t*-test
    c. *F*-test
    d. Correlation with associated *t*-test
    e. Chi-square

6. A researcher claims that USMLE Step 1 scores can be predicted using the following equation:

    $$\text{Score (\%)} = 29 + 0.35X_1 + 1.6X_2 + 3.3X_3$$

    where $X_1 =$ student's IQ, $X_2 =$ number of hours of daily study for the past year, and $X_3 =$ student's GPA at medical school. What statistical technique did the researcher use to arrive at this equation?

    a. Spearman rank-order correlation
    b. Analysis of variance (ANOVA)
    c. Regression
    d. Chi-square
    e. *t*-test

7. A study finds that there is a correlation of $+0.7$ between self-reported work satisfaction and life expectancy in a random sample of 5000 Americans ($p = 0.01$). This means that

    a. work satisfaction is one factor involved in increasing one's life expectancy.
    b. there is a strong statistically significant positive association between work satisfaction and life expectancy.
    c. 70% of people who enjoy their work have an above-average life expectancy.
    d. to live longer, one should try to enjoy one's work.
    e. 70% of the variability in life expectancy in this sample can be accounted for by work satisfaction.

8. In a sample of 200 patients with hypertension who are currently taking antihypertensive medication, it is found that blood pressure and antihypertensive drug dosage correlate $r = -0.3, p < .05$. It is correct to conclude all of the following EXCEPT

    a. the relationship between drug dosage and blood pressure is unlikely to be due to chance.
    b. the relationship between drug dosage and blood pressure is a weak negative one.
    c. although other factors are clearly involved also, drug dosage is one factor causing these patients' blood pressures to be reduced.
    d. drug dosage accounts for 9% of the variation in blood pressures.
    e. it would be possible to make a prediction of a patient's blood pressure from knowledge of their drug dosage by using regression techniques.

9. A study investigates two new drugs that are hypothesized to improve the mean level of recall in patients with Alzheimer's disease. A sample of 1000 patients (500 males, 500 females) are ran-

domly allocated to receive Drug A, Drug B, or a placebo. After 3 months of treatment, all the patients' recall ability is tested. Males' recall is improved by Drug A but is made worse by Drug B, while the converse is true for females. Overall, however, there is no difference between the three treatments or between the two genders. It would be correct to report

a.   no effects.
b.   a drug × gender interaction.
c.   a main effect of age.
d.   a main effect of gender.
e.   a drug × gender interaction and a main effect of gender.

5

Research Methods

Medical researchers typically aim to discover the relationship between one or more events or characteristics (such as being exposed to a toxic substance, having a family history of a certain disease, or taking a certain drug) and others (such as contracting or recovering from a certain illness). All these events or characteristics are called **variables.**

In any type of research, variables may be either **dependent** or **independent.** Independent variables are presumed to be the *causes* of changes in other variables, which are called the dependent variables because they are presumed to *depend* on the values of the independent variables. Research typically attempts to uncover the relationship between independent variables and dependent variables.

EXPERIMENTAL STUDIES

The relationship between dependent and independent variables can be investigated in two ways:

- **Experimental** studies, in which the researcher exercises control over the independent variables, deliberately manipulating them; experimental studies are sometimes called **intervention** studies.

- **Nonexperimental** studies, in which nature is simply allowed to take its course; nonexperimental studies are also called **observational** studies.

For example, in studying the effectiveness of a particular drug for a certain disease, the use or non-use of the drug is the independent variable, and the resulting severity of the disease is the dependent variable, because it is presumed to depend on whether the drug was used or not.

In an *experimental* investigation of the drug's effectiveness, the investigator would intervene, giving the drug to one group of patients but not to another group. In a *nonexperimental* investigation, the researcher would simply observe different patients who had or had not taken the drug in the normal course of events.

As the example suggests, the hallmark of the experimental method is manipulation or intervention. Properly conducted experiments are the most powerful way of establishing cause-and-effect relationships between independent and dependent variables. Nevertheless, they have disadvantages: they may be unethical if they expose subjects to the risk of physical or mental harm, and they are impractical if the cause-effect relationship is one that takes a long time to appear.

If it is hypothesized that it takes 15 years of heavy alcohol drinking to cause cirrhosis of the liver, it would be unethical and impractical to conduct an experiment by administering heavy doses of alcohol to subjects for this length of time to observe the outcome. On the other hand, a researcher could investigate this hypothesis observationally by finding people who have done this in the ordinary course of events.

Clinical trials

The experimental method in medical research commonly takes the form of the **clinical trial,** which attempts to evaluate the effects of a treatment. Clinical trials aim to isolate one factor (such as use of a drug) and examine its contribution to patients' health by holding all other factors as constant as possible. Apart from manipulation or intervention, clinical trials typically have two other characteristics: they utilize **control groups** and involve **randomization.** Hence, they are often termed **randomized controlled clinical trials.**

Control groups

Patients in clinical trials are divided into two general groups:

- the **experimental** group, which is given the treatment under investigation; and

- the **control** group, which is treated in exactly the same way except that it is not given the treatment.

Any difference that appears between the two groups at the end of the study can then be attributed to the treatment under investigation. Control groups therefore help to eliminate alternative explanations for a study's results.

> For example, if a drug eliminates all symptoms of an illness in a group of patients in 1 month, it may be that the symptoms would have disappeared spontaneously over this time even if the drug had not been used. But if a similar control group of patients did not receive the drug and experienced no improvement in their symptoms, this alternative explanation is untenable.

There are two main types of control groups used in medical research:

- The **no-treatment** control group, which is the type used in the previous example: the control group patients receive no treatment at all. This leaves open the possibility that the patients whose symptoms were removed by the drug were responding not to the specific pharmacologic properties of the drug, but to the nonspecific placebo effect that is part of any treatment.

- The **placebo** control group, who are given an inert placebic treatment, allowing the elimination of the explanation that patients in the treatment group who improved were responding to the placebic component of the treatment; so the effectiveness of the drug would have to be attributed to its pharmacologic properties.

In studies of this kind it is obviously important that patients do not know if they are receiving the real drug or the placebo. If patients taking the placebo knew that they were not receiving the real drug, the placebo effect would probably be greatly reduced or eliminated.

It is also important that the physicians or nurses administering the drug and the researchers who assess the patients' outcomes do not know which patients are taking the drug and which are taking the placebo. If they did, this knowledge could cause conscious or unconscious bias that might affect their interactions with and evaluations of the patients. The patients and all those involved with them in the conduct of the experiment should therefore be "blind" as to which patients are in which group. These kinds of studies are therefore called **double-blind** studies. However, it is not always possible to perform a double-blind study.

> For example, in an experiment comparing the effectiveness of a drug versus a surgical procedure, it would be hard to keep the patient "blind" as to which treatment he or she received (although studies have been done in which patients under general anesthesia underwent "sham" surgery). However, it would be possible for the outcome to be measured by a "blind" rater, who might per-

form laboratory tests or interviews with the patient without knowing to which group the patient belonged. Such a study would be called a **single-blind** study.

Under some circumstances, truly controlled experiments may not be possible. In research on the effectiveness of psychotherapy, for example, patients who are placed in a no-treatment control group may well receive help from friends, family, clergy, self-help books, and so on, and would therefore not constitute a true no-treatment control. In this case, the study would be called a **partially controlled** clinical trial.

Controlled experiments pose ethical problems if there is good reason to believe that the treatment under investigation is either a beneficial or a harmful one:

- In the 1950s, experiments on the effects of oxygen on premature babies were opposed on the grounds that the control group would be deprived of a beneficial treatment; later, when it became strongly suspected that excessive oxygen was a cause of a type of blindness (retrolental fibroplasia), similar experiments were opposed because the experimental group might be subjected to a harmful treatment.

- In recent years, a number of drug trials have been cut short because the drug under investigation appeared to be so effective that it was thought unethical to continue depriving the control group patients of the drug (e.g., zidovudine for AIDS, tamoxifen for breast cancer prevention).

Randomization

Randomization means that patients are randomly assigned to different groups (i.e., to the experimental and control groups) to equalize the effects of extraneous variables.

In a controlled trial of a new drug, it would be absurd to assign all the male patients or all the patients with less severe disease to the drug group, and all the females or all the patients with more severe disease to the control group. If this were done, any difference in outcome between the two groups could be attributed to differences between the sexes or pretreatment severities of the disease in the two groups rather than to the drug itself. In this kind of situation, patient gender and disease severity are called **confounding variables,** because they contribute differently and inextricably to the two groups. To avoid confounding effects, patients are normally assigned randomly to the two groups, so that the different independent variables (in this case, gender, disease severity, and receiving the drug) are not systematically related.

Allocating patients randomly to the different experimental groups guards against bias. True randomization means that the groups should be similar with respect to gender, disease severity, age, occupation, and any other variable that may differentially affect response to the experimental intervention.

Matching

Randomization cannot *guarantee* that the experimental and control groups are similar in all important ways. An alternative way of doing this is to use **matching:** each patient in the experimental group is paired with a patient in the control group who matches him or her closely on all relevant characteristics. If gender, race, and age were important factors influencing the course of the disease being studied, each experimental patient would be matched with a control patient of the same gender, race, and age. Thus, any resulting differences between the two groups could not be attributed to differences in gender, race, or age.

Stratified randomization

This is a combination of randomization and matching techniques. The population under study is first divided, or **stratified,** into subgroups that are internally homogeneous with respect to the important factors (e.g., race, age, disease severity). Equal numbers of patients from each subgroup are then randomly allocated to the experimental and control groups. The two groups are therefore similar, but their exact membership is still a result of randomization.

Experimental designs

In the studies mentioned so far, comparisons are made between patients (or subjects) in one group and patients in the other group; these studies are therefore called **between-subjects** designs. Alternatively, each patient can be used as his or her *own* control, which means that comparisons are being made *within* each subject, a **within-subjects** design, and the control group is a **same-subject** control group. This method solves the problem of achieving comparability between the control and experimental groups.

A common type of research using the within-subjects approach is the **crossover** design. Here half the patients receive the placebo for a period, followed by the experimental treatment; the other half receive the treatment first, then the placebo. If there is a danger of a "carryover" effect (for example, if the treatment is a drug that may continue to have some effect after it is withdrawn), then there can be a **washout** period in between the drug and placebo phases, during which no treatment is given.

Figure 5–1 illustrates a crossover design with washout. One group of patients receives the drug for 1 month and then "crosses over" to receive the placebo after 1 month's washout. The other group follows this pattern in reverse order. The efficacy of the drug is determined by comparing the effects of the drug and placebo *within each patient*. This kind of design is also called a **repeated measures** design, because the measurements (of the dependent variable, such as the severity of the patients' symptoms) are repeated within each patient at different times, and results are analyzed by comparing the measurements that have been repeated on each patient.

NONEXPERIMENTAL STUDIES

Nonexperimental (or observational) studies fall into two general classes: **descriptive studies** and **analytic studies.**

Descriptive studies

These aim to describe the occurrence and distribution of disease or other phenomena. They do not try to offer explanations or test a theory or a hypothesis. They merely attempt to generate a description of the frequency of the disease or other phenomenon of interest according to the places, times, and people involved. These studies will use descriptive statistics but not inferential statistics.

Descriptive studies are often the first method used to study a particular disease—hence, they are also called **exploratory studies**—and they may serve to generate hypotheses for analytic studies to test. Well-

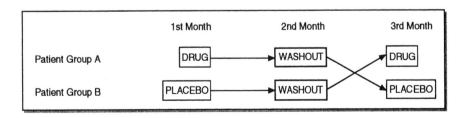

Figure 5-1

known examples of modern descriptive studies include those of Legionnaire's disease following its first recognized outbreak in 1976, and early studies of AIDS showing that male homosexuals, intravenous drug abusers, and persons with hemophilia were at risk. In both these cases, the true nature of the disease was unknown at the time, but the findings of descriptive studies generated useful hypotheses.

Analytic studies

These aim to test hypotheses or to provide explanations about a disease or other phenomena—hypotheses or explanations that are often drawn from earlier descriptive studies. They therefore use inferential statistics to test hypotheses.

Descriptive and analytic studies are not always entirely distinguishable. For example, a large-scale descriptive study may provide such clear data that it may provide an answer to questions or give clear support to a particular hypothesis.

Nonexperimental designs

Descriptive or analytic studies use one of four principal research designs: they may be **cohort studies, case-control studies, case series studies,** or **prevalence surveys.**

Cohort studies

Cohort studies focus on factors related to the development of a disease. A **cohort** (a group of people) that does *not* have the disease of interest is selected and then observed for an extended period. Some members of the cohort will already have been exposed to a suspected risk factor for the disease, and others will eventually become exposed; by following them all, the relationship between the risk factors and the eventual outcomes can be seen. This kind of study therefore allows the incidence and natural history of a disease to be studied.

Cohort studies may be loosely termed **follow-up** or **longitudinal** studies because they follow people over a prolonged period, tracing any changes through repeated observation. They are also called **prospective** studies because people are followed forward from a particular point in time, so the researcher is "prospecting" or looking for data about events that are yet to happen. In addition, cohort studies are sometimes called **incidence** studies because they look for the incidence of new cases of the disease over time.

> A famous example of a cohort study is the Framingham Study, which was begun in 1949. This started with a cohort of more than 5000 people in Framingham, Massachusetts, who were free of coronary heart disease (CHD). The individuals in the cohort were reexamined every 2 years for more than 30 years. This study succeeded in identifying the major physical risk factors for CHD.

Another example is the Western Collaborative Group Study (WCGS), which followed a cohort of more than 5000 heart disease-free California males for 7 years, showing that type A personality was strongly associated with increased risk of CHD. (This study has subsequently been extended to a 21-year follow-up, with somewhat contradictory results.)

 Cohort studies have a number of significant advantages:

1. When a true experiment cannot be conducted (whether for ethical or practical reasons), cohort studies are the best form of investigation; their findings are often extremely valuable.

2. They are the only method that can establish the absolute risk of contracting a disease, and they help to answer one of the most clinically relevant questions: if someone is exposed to a certain suspected risk factor, is that person more likely to contract the disease? Cohort studies may also reveal the existence of protective factors, such as exercise and diet.

3. Because cohort studies are prospective, the assessment of risk factors in these studies is unbiased by the outcome. If the Framingham Study were retrospective, for example, people's recollection of their diet and smoking habits could have been biased by the fact that they already have CHD (this effect is known as **recall bias**). In addition, the chronologic relationship between the risk factors and the disease is clear; if the WCGS were retrospective, it might be unclear whether people developed a type A personality style *after* contracting CHD, rather than before.

4. For the individuals in a cohort who ultimately contract the disease of interest, data concerning their exposure to suspected risk factors have already been collected. However, in a retrospective study this may not be possible. Again, if the Framingham Study were retrospective, it might have been impossible to obtain accurate information about the diet and smoking habits of people who had already died. If the WCGS were retrospective, it would have been difficult if not impossible to assess the personality of people who had already died. Other types of studies are often unable to include people who die of the disease in question— often the most important people to study.

5. Information about suspected risk factors collected in cohort studies can be used to examine the relationship between these risk factors and *many* diseases; therefore, a study designed as an analytic investigation of one disease may simultaneously serve as a valuable descriptive study of several other diseases.

Cohort studies have some important disadvantages:

1. They are time-consuming, laborious, and expensive to conduct; members of the cohort must be followed for a long time (often for many years) before a sufficient number of them get the disease of interest. It will often be very expensive and difficult to keep track of a large number of people for several years, and it may be many years before results are produced, especially in the case of diseases that take a long time to appear after exposure to a risk factor.

2. They may be impractical for rare diseases. For example, if 1 case of a disease occurs in every 10,000 people, then 100,000 people will have to be followed for 10 cases to eventually appear. However, if a particular cohort with a high rate of the disease exists, such as an occupational cohort, a disease that is rare in the general population can still be studied by this method. Classic examples of this include studies of scrotal cancer among chimney sweeps and bladder cancer among dye workers..

Case-control studies

Whereas cohort studies examine people who are initially free of the disease of interest, **case-control** studies compare people who *do* have the disease (the cases) with otherwise similar people who *do not* have the disease (the controls).

Case-control studies start with the outcome, or dependent variable (the presence or absence of the disease). They then look *back* into the past for possible independent variables that may have caused the disease, to see if a possible risk factor was present more frequently in cases than controls. Hence, they are also called **retrospective** studies.

One classic exploratory case-control study uncovered the relationship between maternal exposure to diethylstilbestrol (DES) and carcinoma of the vagina in young women (Herbst *et al.*, 1971). Eight patients with this rare cancer were each compared with four matched cancer-free controls. Looking back at their individual and maternal histories, no significant differences appeared between the cases and the controls on a wide range of variables, but it was found that mothers of seven of the eight cases had taken DES in early pregnancy, 15 to 20 years earlier, while none of the 32 controls' mothers had done so.

Case-control studies offer some significant advantages:

1.   They can be performed fairly quickly and cheaply (especially in comparison with cohort studies), even for rare diseases or diseases that take a long time to appear (as the vaginal carcinoma example shows). Because of this, case-control studies are the most important way of investigating rare diseases and are typically used in the early exploration of a disease.

2.   They require comparatively few subjects.

3.   They allow multiple potential causes of a disease to be investigated.

Case-control studies also have a number of disadvantages and are particularly subject to bias:

1.   People's recall of their past behaviors or risk factor exposure may be biased by the fact that they now have the disease.

2.   The only cases that can be investigated are people who have been identified and diagnosed; undiagnosed or asymptomatic cases are missed by this kind of study. People who have already died of the disease cannot be questioned about their past behaviors and exposure to risk factors.

3.   Selecting a comparable control group is a difficult task that relies entirely on the researcher's judgment.

4.   Case-control studies cannot determine the rates or the risk of the disease in exposed and nonexposed people.

5.   They cannot prove a cause-effect relationship.

Case series studies

A **case series** simply describes the presentation of a disease in a number of patients. It does not follow the patients for a period, and it uses no control or comparison group. Therefore, it cannot establish a cause-effect relationship, and its validity is entirely a matter for the reader to decide. A report that 8 of a series of 10 patients with a certain disease have a history of exposure to a particular risk factor may be judged to be extremely useful or almost worthless.

Despite these serious shortcomings, case series studies are commonly used to present new information about patients with rare diseases, and they may stimulate new hypotheses. They can be done by almost any clinician who carefully observes and records patient information. A **case report** is a special form of case series in which only one patient is described—this too may be very valuable or virtually worthless.

Prevalence surveys

A **prevalence survey** or **community survey** is a survey of a whole population. It assesses the proportion of people with a certain disease (this is the **prevalence** of the disease; see Fig. 6–1) and examines the relationship between the disease and other characteristics of the population. Because prevalence surveys are based on a single examination of the population at a particular point in time and do not follow the population over time, they are also called **cross-sectional** studies, in distinction to longitudinal (cohort) studies.

Prevalence surveys are common in the medical literature. Examples include a study of the prevalence of CHD in a community, which could be compared with a different community with different dietary or exercise habits. Another example is a study examining the prevalence of respiratory disease in a city, which could then be compared with another city with lower levels of cigarette consumption or air pollution.

Prevalence surveys suffer from a number of disadvantages:

1. Because they look at existing cases of a disease, and not at the occurrence of new cases, they are likely to over-represent chronic diseases and under-represent acute diseases.

2. They may be unusable for acute diseases, which few people suffered from at the moment they were surveyed.

3. People with some types of disease may leave the community, or may be institutionalized, causing them to be excluded from the survey.

Findings of prevalence surveys must be interpreted cautiously; the mere fact that two variables (such as high fish intake and reduced coronary disease) are associated does not mean that they are causally related.

Although they are expensive and laborious, prevalence surveys are common because they can produce valuable data about a wide range of diseases, behaviors, and characteristics. These data can be used to generate hypotheses for more analytic studies to examine.

EXERCISES

Questions 1–7

Select the single, best answer to the following questions.

1. Which of the following research methods studies only people who are initially free of the disease of interest?

a. A case-control study
b. A case series study
c. A prevalence survey
d. A cohort study
e. A clinical trial

2. What is the purpose of a control group in an experimental study?

a. It permits an ethical alternative for patients who do not wish to be subjected to an experimental treatment.
b. It allows larger numbers of patients to be used, thus increasing the power of the statistical techniques used.
c. It helps to eliminate alternative explanations for the results of the study.
d. It reduces the likelihood of making a type II error in hypothesis testing.

3. What is the purpose of randomization in a clinical trial?

a. To equalize the effects of extraneous variables, thus guarding against bias.
b. To allow inferential statistics to be used.

c. To guard against placebo effects.
d. To guard against ethical problems in the allocation of patients to experimental and control groups.

4. When a controlled experiment cannot be performed, which of the following is the best alternative?

a. Case-control study
b. Cohort study
c. Case series
d. Retrospective study
e. Prevalence survey

5. A pharmaceutical company develops a new antihypertensive drug. A sample of 24 hypertensive patients, randomly selected from a large population of hypertensive people, are randomly divided into 2 groups of 12. One group is given the new drug over a period of 1 month; the other group is given a placebo according to the same schedule. Neither the patients nor the treating physicians are aware of which patients are in which group. At the end of the month, measurements are made of the patients' blood pressures. This study

a. is a randomized controlled clinical trial.
b. uses a crossover design.
c. is a single-blind experiment.
d. is a prospective study.
d. is a case-control study.

6. A researcher wishes to test the effects of a new drug. He gives 100 male patients the drug, and gives 100 female patients a placebo on the same daily schedule. After 1 month he compares the reduction in symptoms experienced by the drug and placebo groups. What is the most important thing that this researcher should have done to improve the validity of his findings?

a. Used a double-blind design.
b. Used a prospective design.
c. Used randomization.
d. Used dependent and independent variables.
e. Performed an experimental study instead.

7. A study compared 150 children with a particular disease with 300 disease-free children to examine past experiences that may contribute to the development of the illness. What kind of study is this?

a. Cohort
b. Controlled clinical trial
c. Prospective
d. Case series
e. Case-control

Questions 8–15

The following questions are matching. Choose the one best answer to each question.

a. Cohort studies
b. Case-control studies
c. Case series studies
d. Prevalence surveys
e. Controlled clinical trials

8. Also known as a retrospective study.

9. Suitable for seeking the cause of very rare diseases.

10. Are typically very expensive and may take several years to produce results.

11. Are the only method of establishing the absolute risk of contracting a disease.

12. Commonly uses random allocation of participants to different groups.

13. Used to help determine the cause of a disease, can usually be performed quickly and cheaply, requires few subjects, and presents no significant ethical problems.

14. The most powerful way of establishing cause-and-effect relationships.

15. Also known as a prospective study.

6

Statistics in Epidemiology

Epidemiology is the study of the distribution, determinants, and dynamics of health and disease in groups of people in relation to their environment and ways of living. The basic statistical measures in epidemiology are **rates** and **measures of risk.**

RATES

All rates consist of a numerator (usually the number of people with a particular condition) and a denominator (usually the number of people at risk), and they usually specify a unit of time. The most important rates are **incidence** and **prevalence** (which are both measures of **morbidity**), **mortality,** and **case-fatality.**

Incidence

The **incidence** of a disease is the number of new cases occurring in a particular time period, such as 1 year. The incidence rate is therefore the ratio of new cases of the disease to the total number of people at risk:

$$\text{Incidence rate} = \frac{\text{number of new cases of the disease}}{\text{total number of people at risk}} \text{ per unit of time}$$

The incidence rate is often stated per 100,000 of the population at risk, or as a percentage. Incidence rates are found by the use of cohort studies, which are therefore sometimes also known as incidence studies (see Chapter 5). For example, if the incidence of shingles in a community is 2000 per 100,000 per annum, this tells us that in 1 year, 2% of the population experiences an episode of shingles.

Prevalence

The **prevalence** of a disease is the number of people affected by it at a particular moment in time. The prevalence rate is therefore the ratio of the number of people with the disease to the total number of people at risk:

$$\text{Prevalence rate} = \frac{\text{number of people with the disease}}{\text{total number of people at risk}} \text{ at a particular time}$$

Like incidence rates, prevalence rates are often stated per 100,000 people, or as a percentage. They are generally found by prevalence surveys. For example, at a given time 170 of every 100,000 people (0.17%) in a community might be suffering from shingles.

Prevalence is an appropriate measure of the burden of a relatively stable chronic condition (such as hypertension or diabetes). However, it is not generally appropriate for acute illnesses, as it depends on the average duration of the disease—it is of little value to speak of the prevalence of pulmonary emboli or myocardial infarctions.

Prevalence is equal to the *incidence multiplied by the average duration of the disease*, so an increased prevalence rate may merely reflect increased duration of an acute illness, rather than suggesting that members of the population are at greater risk of contracting the disease.

The incidence and prevalence rates of shingles given in the above examples suggest that the average episode of this illness lasts approximately 1 month, as the prevalence is one-twelfth of the annual incidence. If a new treatment cut the duration of an episode of shingles in half, to 2 weeks, but did nothing to prevent shingles from occurring, the incidence would not change but the prevalence at any given time would be cut in half:

Before new treatment:

$$\text{Prevalence} = \text{annual incidence} \times \text{average duration (in years)}$$
$$= 2\% \times 1/12$$
$$= 0.17\%$$

After new treatment:

$$\text{Prevalence} = \text{annual incidence} \times \text{average duration (in years)}$$
$$= 2\% \times 1/24$$
$$= 0.085\%$$

Incidence and prevalence are both measures of **morbidity,** or the rate of illness.

Mortality

Mortality is the number of deaths. The mortality rate is the ratio of the number of people dying (whether of a specific disease or of all causes) to the total number of people at risk:

$$\text{Mortality rate} = \frac{\text{total number of deaths}}{\text{total number of people at risk}} \text{ per unit of time}$$

Like incidence and prevalence, mortality rates may be expressed as a percentage, or the number of deaths per 1000 or 100,000 people, typically per annum. Mortality is actually a special form of incidence in which the event in question is death rather than contracting a disease. Mortality figures are likely to be more accurate than incidence figures, because deaths are always recorded whereas episodes of illness are not. However, accurate records of causes of death are often unavailable, and mortality rates will not reflect the total burden of illness except in the case of diseases that are always fatal.

 ### The "epidemiologist's bathtub"

The relationships between incidence, prevalence, and mortality in any disease can be visualized with the aid of the "epidemiologist's bathtub," shown in Figure 6–1.

- The flow of water through the faucet into the bathtub is analogous to incidence, representing the arrival of new cases of the disease.

- The level of water in the tub represents the prevalence, or number of cases of the disease existing at any given point in time.

- The flow of water out through the drain represents mortality.

- The evaporation of water represents either cure or a natural progression to recovery.

Alzheimer's disease provides an example of the application of the "bathtub." The incidence (inflow

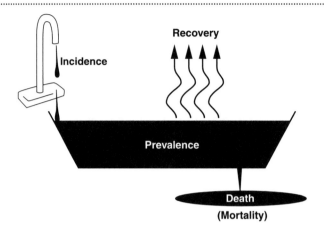

Figure 6-1

of water) of Alzheimer's disease is roughly constant, and modern medicine is able to keep Alzheimer's patients alive for longer, thus reducing the mortality rate from the disease (partially blocking the drain). However, because there is no cure for the disease, and it never progresses to recovery, the result is clearly an increased prevalence (increased water level)—which is apparent in the United States today. This picture is also broadly true of AIDS in the United States.

Case fatality

The **case fatality rate** (CFR) is the ratio of the number of people dying in a particular episode of a disease to the total number of episodes of the disease, expressed as a percentage:

$$\text{CFR} = \frac{\text{total number of people dying in an episode of the disease}}{\text{total number of episodes of the disease}} \times 100$$

The CFR is a measure of the prognosis, in terms of life or death, for an episode of a given disease, because it shows the likelihood of one episode or occurrence of it resulting in death. It is used to follow the effectiveness of treatments over time or in different places (e.g., what is the CFR of acute myocardial infarction or pulmonary embolism in a given hospital or community?).

Attack rates

The **attack rate** is the ratio of the number of people contracting a particular disease to the total number of people at risk, expressed as a percentage:

$$\text{Attack rate} = \frac{\text{number of people contracting a disease}}{\text{total number of people at risk}} \times 100$$

For example, if 1000 people eat at a barbecue at which contaminated food is served, and 300 of these people become sick, the attack rate is $(300/1000) \times 100 = 30\%$.

Attack rates are useful in attempting to deduce the source of an epidemic. To take the barbecue example, different people will have eaten different combinations of foods. Table 6–1 shows the attack rates for each food.

Table 6-1

Food	Number who ate	Number who got sick	Attack rate
Chicken only	100	25	25%
Ribs only	80	10	12.5%
Cole slaw only	20	7	35%
Chicken & ribs only	200	18	9%
Chicken & ribs & cole slaw	600	240	40%
Overall	1000	300	30%

The source of the illness can be deduced by inspecting the table for the maximum difference between any two attack rates. The largest difference between any two attack rates is 31%, which is the difference between the lowest rate, 9% (in those who ate the chicken and ribs only), and the highest rate, 40% (in those who ate the chicken, ribs, and cole slaw). The implication is therefore that the cole slaw is the source.

Adjustment of rates

Researchers may want to compare rates across different populations (e.g., to compare the incidence of a disease in two cities or countries). However, if the populations differ significantly on one or more factors that are relevant to the illness in question, the comparison will be biased.

> For example, a researcher wants to compare the prevalence of AIDS in two cities of equal size. City A has a large proportion of elderly people, whereas city B does not—so it would not be surprising if city A had a lower prevalence of AIDS than city B. However, due to the confounding effects of the different age structures of the two cities' populations, this prevalence rate alone tells the researcher nothing about any real underlying difference in the prevalence of AIDS in the two cities.

This biasing influence of a confounding variable such as age can be removed by the technique of **adjustment** (or **standardization**) **of rates.** This involves calculating rates for the two populations as if they were both the same in terms of the factors (such as age) that are relevant to the disease, so that their rates of the disease can be compared. This kind of process of adjustment (or standardization) can be done not only for age, but also for any other relevant factor that differs substantially between two populations that are being compared. Adjustment can be made for two or more factors simultaneously; for example, if city A had many more IV drug abusers than city B, this difference could also be adjusted for. Mortality rates are commonly standardized, producing a statistic called **standardized mortality ratio** (SMR). USMLE will not require knowledge of the mathematics of adjustment of rates.

MEASUREMENT OF RISK

Information about the risk of contracting a disease is of great value in medicine. The knowledge that something is a risk factor for a disease can be used to help in:

- preventing the disease,

- predicting its future incidence and prevalence,

- diagnosing it (diagnostic suspicions will be aroused if it is known that a patient was exposed to the risk factor), and

- establishing the cause of a disease of unknown etiology.

Absolute risk

The fundamental measure of risk is incidence. The incidence of a disease is, in fact, the **absolute risk** of contracting it. For example, if the incidence of a disease is 10 per 1000 people per annum, then the absolute risk of a person actually contracting it is also 10 per 1000 per annum, or 1% per annum.

It is useful to go beyond absolute risk and to compare the incidence of a disease in different groups of people to find out if exposure to a suspected risk factor (such as smoking cigarettes) increases the risk of contracting a certain disease (such as lung cancer). A number of different comparisons of risk can be made, including **relative risk, attributable risk,** and the **odds ratio.** All these are called **measures of effect**—they measure the effect of being exposed to a risk factor on the risk of contracting a disease.

The ideal way of determining the effect of a risk factor is by a controlled experiment, but this is rarely ethical. The best alternative is the cohort (prospective) study, in which the incidence of disease in exposed and nonexposed people can be observed directly.

One of the main goals of these studies (such as the Framingham Study and the Western Group Collaborative Study, described briefly in Chapter 5) is to find the extent to which the risk of contracting the disease is increased by exposure to the risk factor. The two measures that show this are **relative risk** and **attributable risk.**

Relative risk

Relative risk states by how many times exposure to the risk factor increases the risk of contracting the disease. It is therefore the ratio of the incidence of the disease among exposed persons to the incidence of the disease among unexposed persons:

$$\text{Relative risk} = \frac{\text{incidence of the disease among persons exposed to the risk factor}}{\text{incidence of the disease among persons not exposed to the risk factor}}$$

As an example, Table 6–2 reports the results of a hypothetical cohort study of lung cancer in which 1008 heavy smokers and 1074 nonsmokers were followed for a number of years. The incidence of lung cancer over the total time period of the study among people exposed to the risk factor (heavy cigarette smoking) is 283/1008, or .28 (28%), while the incidence among those not exposed is 64/1074, or .06 (6%).

The relative risk is therefore .28/.06, or 4.67, showing that people who smoked cigarettes heavily were 4.67 times more likely to contract lung cancer than were nonsmokers. (Note that this not a measure of *absolute* risk—it states nothing about the likelihood of heavy smokers contracting cancer in absolute terms.)

Because relative risk is a ratio of risks, it is sometimes called the **risk ratio,** or **morbidity ratio.** In the case of outcomes involving death, rather than just disease, it may also be called the **mortality ratio.**

Many clinical trials report **relative risk *reductions*** due to the use of a drug; relative risk reduction is equal to 1 − relative risk:

Table 6-2

RISK	Lung Cancer	No Lung Cancer	Total
		DISEASE OUTCOME	
Exposed (heavy smokers)	283	725	1008
Nonexposed (nonsmokers)	64	1010	1074
Total	347	1735	2082

Relative risk reduction = 1 − relative risk

Relative risk reduction figures may be misleading if not understood properly. This can be illustrated by the well-known West of Scotland Coronary Prevention (WOSCOPS) study (Shepherd *et al.*, 1995):

> This study was a double-blind randomized clinical trial in which approximately 6000 men with elevated cholesterol levels were randomly assigned to groups taking either a placebo or the cholesterol-lowering drug pravastatin for an average of 4.9 years.

There were 73 deaths from cardiovascular causes in the placebo group (3293 men); the cardiovascular mortality rate was therefore $73/3293 = 0.022$ (2.2%) in this group. In the pravastatin group (3302 men), there 50 deaths from cardiovascular causes, giving a mortality rate of $50/3302 = 0.015$, or 1.5%. The relative risk of death in those given the drug is $1.5/2.2 = 0.68$, so the relative risk reduction is 1 − 0.68 = 0.32, or 32%—showing that an impressive 32% of cardiovascular deaths were prevented by the drug.

However, the **absolute risk reduction** is 2.2% − 1.5% = 0.7%—a far less impressive-sounding figure, showing that of all men given the drug for 4.9 years, 0.7% of them were saved from a cardiovascular death.

Absolute risk reduction allows calculation of another statistic that is of clinical importance. If 0.7% of patients were saved by the drug, this implies that $(100/0.7) = 143$ patients would have to be treated to save 1 life. This figure is called the **number needed to treat,** or **NNT,** and it allows the effectiveness of different treatments to be compared:

Number needed to treat = 1/absolute risk reduction

The NNT allows a further calculation—the cost of saving one life with the treatment. WOSCOPS showed that 143 men needed to be treated for 4.9 years (58 months) to save 1 life; as the dose of pravastatin used in the study costs approximately $100 per month, it would cost $100 × 58 = $5800 to treat one man for this length of time. It would therefore cost $5800 × 143 = $829,400 to prevent one cardiovascular death over this period. This gives a very different perspective on the value of a treatment than the statement that it reduces the risk of death by 32%. Similar analyses can be performed easily for almost any clinical trial in the literature.

Attributable risk

The attributable risk is the *additional* incidence of a disease that is attributable to the risk factor in question. It is equal to the incidence of the disease in exposed persons minus the incidence of the disease in nonexposed persons.

In the example of lung cancer and smokers, the attributable risk is .28 − .06, or .22 (22%)—in other words, of the 28% incidence of lung cancer among the heavy smokers in this study, 22% is attributable to smoking. The other 6% is the "background" incidence of the disease—its incidence among those not exposed to this particular risk factor. Attributable risk is sometimes called **risk difference,** because it is the difference in the risks or incidences of the disease between the two groups of people.

Odds ratio

Relative risk and attributable risk both require the use of cohort (prospective) studies, as shown previously. As noted in Chapter 5, cohort studies are generally expensive and time-consuming and are therefore often impractical.

A common alternative is to use a case-control (retrospective) study, which compares people *with* the disease (cases) with otherwise similar people *without* the disease (controls), attempting to look back into the past to see if a possible risk factor is found more frequently among the cases than the controls (see Chapter 5). If the proportion of people who were exposed to the possible risk factor is greater among the cases, then the risk factor is implicated as a cause of the disease. The **odds ratio** (or **relative odds**) is a measure of these relative proportions—it is the ratio of the odds that a case was exposed to the odds that a control was exposed:

$$\text{Odds ratio} = \frac{\text{odds that a case was exposed to the risk factor}}{\text{odds that a control was exposed to the risk factor}}$$

Because the proportion of people in the study who do have the disease is determined by the researcher's choice, and not by the actual proportion in the population, case-control studies cannot determine the incidence or prevalence of a disease, so they *cannot determine the risk of contracting a disease*. The odds ratio must therefore be used instead of relative risk when analyzing case-control data instead of cohort data.

For example, the hypothetical data that were used to illustrate the calculation of relative risk in Table 6–2 can be used, but now it will be assumed that these data were generated by a case-control study in which history of prior exposure to the risk factor (cigarette smoking) was compared between 347 cases (with lung cancer) and 1735 controls (without lung cancer).

As defined previously, the odds ratio is the ratio of the odds that a case was exposed to the odds that a control was exposed; it can be shown[1] that this is equal to

$$\frac{\text{number of cases exposed to risk factor } (A) \times \text{number of controls not exposed } (D)}{\text{number of controls exposed to risk factor } (B) \times \text{number of cases not exposed } (C)}$$

Table 6-3 shows that:

283 of the cases were exposed to the risk factor (A)

725 of the controls were exposed to the risk factor (B)

64 of the cases were not exposed to the risk factor (C)

1010 of the controls were not exposed to the risk factor (D)

The odds ratio is, therefore, $\dfrac{283 \times 1010}{725 \times 64} = \dfrac{285830}{46400} = 6.16$

Table 6-3

| | DISEASE OUTCOME | | |
RISK	Lung Cancer (Cases)	No Lung Cancer	Total
Exposed (heavy smokers)	283 (A)	725 (B)	1008
Nonexposed (nonsmokers)	64 (C)	1010 (D)	1074
Total	347	1736	2082

In other words, among the people studied, a person with lung cancer was 6.16 times more likely to have been exposed to the risk factor (cigarette smoking) than was a person without lung cancer.

An odds ratio of 1 indicates that a person with the disease is no more likely to have been exposed to the risk factor than is a person without the disease, suggesting that the risk factor is not related to the disease. An odds ratio of less than 1 indicates that a person with the disease is *less* likely to have been exposed to the risk factor than is a person without the disease, implying that the risk factor may actually be a *protective* factor against the disease.

In some ways the odds ratio is similar to the relative risk: both figures demonstrate the strength of the association between the risk factor and the disease, albeit in different ways. As a result of their similarities, the odds ratio is sometimes called **estimated relative risk**—it provides a reasonably good estimate of relative risk *provided* that the incidence of the disease is low (which is usually true of chronic diseases), and that the cases and controls examined in the study are representative of people with and without the disease in the population.

NOTE

The derivation of this is as follows. Referring to the cells in Table 6-3, the odds that a case was exposed are $\dfrac{A/(A + C)}{C/(A + C)} = A/C$.

The odds that a control was exposed are $\dfrac{B/(B + D)}{D/(B + D)} = B/D$.

The ratio of these odds is $\dfrac{A/C}{B/D}$.

which, when cross-multiplied, becomes $\dfrac{A \times D}{B \times C}$.

EXERCISES

Questions 1–3

Select the single, best answer to the following questions.

1. A new treatment reduces the average duration of an illness, but it does not alter the number of new cases or the number of people dying of the disease. It will therefore

    a. decrease the prevalence of the disease.
    b. increase the prevalence of the disease.
    c. decrease the incidence of the disease.
    d. increase the incidence of the disease.
    e. leave both incidence and prevalence unchanged.

2. In a 5-year period, there were 160 cases of pulmonary embolism recorded in a hospital. Twenty of these cases resulted in death. The case-fatality rate is therefore

    a. $160 - 20 = 140$.
    b. $160 \times 20 = 3200$.
    c. $(160 \times 20)/5 = 640$.
    d. $20/160 = 0.125$ or 12.5%.
    e. $160/20 = 8$.

3. Improved prevention of an acute, nonfatal disease is likely to

    a. decrease the prevalence of the disease.
    b. increase the prevalence of the disease.
    c. decrease the incidence of the disease.
    d. increase the incidence of the disease.
    e. decrease both the incidence and prevalence of the disease.

Questions 4–9

The following questions refer to Table 6–4, which shows the number of cases of breast cancer occurring in a randomized clinical trial of a new drug designed to prevent the disease. In this study, 1000 healthy women between the ages of 60 and 65 were given the drug and 1000 were given the placebo for 5 years.

4. What is the absolute risk (over the 5 years duration of the study) of getting breast cancer for patients in the placebo group?

    a. 4%
    b. 1.6
    c. 24
    d. 67.5%
    e. 0.4

Table 6-4

TREATMENT	DISEASE OUTCOME	
	Breast cancer	No breast cancer
Placebo	40	960
Drug	10	990

5. What is the absolute risk (over the 5 years duration of the study) of getting breast cancer for patients in the drug group?

a. 30
b. 25%
c. 1%
d. 4
e. 0.5

6. What is the relative risk reduction of breast cancer attributable to the drug?

a. 25%
b. 50%
c. 75%
d. 100%
e. 150%

7. What is the absolute risk reduction in breast cancer attributable to the drug?

a. 1%
b. 2%
c. 3%
d. 4%

8. What is the number needed to treat (NNT) to prevent one case of breast cancer?

a. 2
b. 3
c. 4
d. 33.3
e. Cannot be calculated from the information given.

9. If the drug cost $100 per month, what would be the cost of preventing 1 case of breast cancer in this 5-year study?

a. $1200
b. $6000
c. $20,000
d. $200,000
e. $330,000

7

Statistics in Medical Decision Making

Medical decision making often involves using various kinds of tests or numeric data. Any physician using a diagnostic test—whether a physical test or a laboratory test performed on an individual patient, or a screening test being used on a whole population—will want to know how good the test is.

This is a complex question, as the qualities and characteristics of tests can be evaluated in several important ways. To assess the quality of a diagnostic test, it is necessary as a minimum to know its

- validity and reliability,

- sensitivity and specificity, and

- positive and negative predictive values.

When using quantitative test results—such as measurements of fasting glucose, serum cholesterol, and hematocrit levels—the physician will need to know the **accuracy** and **precision** of the measurement as well as the **normal reference** values for the variable in question.

VALIDITY

The validity of a test is the extent to which it actually tests what it claims to test—in other words, how closely its results correspond to the real state of affairs. The validity of a diagnostic or screening test is, therefore, its ability to show which individuals have the disease in question and which do not. To be truly valid, a test should be highly sensitive, specific (see section on Sensitivity and Specificity in this chapter), and unbiased. Quantitatively, the validity of a diagnostic or screening test is the proportion of all test results that are correct, as determined by comparison with an accepted standard (sometimes called the **gold standard**) which is known to be totally correct.

Validity is synonymous with accuracy. As stated in Chapter 2, the accuracy of a figure or measurement is the degree to which it is immune from systematic error or bias. To the extent that a measurement or test result is free from systematic error or bias, it is accurate and valid. When assessing the validity of a research study as a whole, two kinds of validity are involved:

- **Internal validity:** are the results of the study valid for the population of patients who were actually studied?

- **External validity:** are the results of the study valid for other patients?

For example, a study of 1000 white American women might demonstrate that calcium supplements are beneficial in preventing osteoporosis. The study, if properly performed on a representative random sample of white American women, would be internally valid. However, what does it tell a physician who wants to prevent osteoporosis in a patient population that may come from a different demographic background?

RELIABILITY

Reliability is synonymous with repeatability and reproducibility—it is the level of agreement between repeated measurements of the same variable. Hence, it is also called **test-retest reliability**. In the case of a test of a stable variable, it can be quantified in terms of the correlation between measurements made at different times. This is the test's "reliability coefficient."

Reliability corresponds to precision, defined in Chapter 2 as the degree to which a figure is immune from random variation. A test that is affected very little by random variation will obviously produce very similar results when it is used to measure a stable variable at different times. A reliable test is therefore a consistent, stable, and dependable one.

The reliability or repeatability of a test influences the extent to which a single measurement may be taken as a definitive guide for making a diagnosis. In the case of a highly reliable test, one measurement alone may be sufficient to allow a physician to diagnose with confidence; however, if the test is unreliable in any way, this may not be possible. The inherent instability of many biomedical variables (such as blood pressure) often makes it necessary to repeat a measurement at different times and to use the mean of these results to obtain a reliable measurement and make a confident diagnosis.

In practice, neither validity nor reliability is usually in question in routine hospital laboratory testing. Standard laboratory tests have been carefully validated, and careful quality control procedures in the laboratory ensure reliability.

A test or measurement may be reliable or precise without necessarily being valid or accurate. For example, it would be possible to measure the circumference of a person's skull with great reliability and precision, but this would certainly not constitute a valid assessment of the person's intelligence.

Bias may also cause a reliable and precise measurement to be invalid. A laboratory balance, for example, may weigh very precisely, with very little variation between repeated weighings of the same object. However, if it has not been zeroed properly, all its measurements may be 3 mg too high, causing all its results to be biased and hence inaccurate and invalid.

Conversely, a measurement may be valid, yet unreliable. In medicine this is often due to the inherent instability of the variable being measured. Repeated measurements of a patient's blood pressure may vary considerably; yet if all these measurements cluster around one figure, the findings as a whole may accurately represent the true state of affairs (e.g., that a patient is hypertensive).

REFERENCE VALUES

No matter how high the quality of a set of measurements, they do not in themselves permit the physician to make a diagnosis, even if they are both valid and reliable. To make a diagnosis, the physician must have some idea of the measurement's range of values among normal, healthy people. This range is called the **normal range** or **reference range,** and the limits of this range are the reference values that the physician will use to interpret the values obtained from the patient. (The range between the reference values is sometimes called the **reference interval**).

How can a valid set of reference values be established? The "normal range" or "reference range" of a biomedical variable is often arbitrarily defined as the middle 95% of the normal (or Gaussian) distribution—in other words, the population mean plus or minus two standard deviations (explained in Chapter 2). The limits of this range, derived from a healthy population, are therefore the "reference values." The assumptions being made here are that:

- the 95% of the population that lie within this range are "normal," whereas the 5% beyond it are "abnormal" or "pathologic," and

- the "normal range" for a particular biomedical variable (e.g., serum cholesterol) can be obtained by measuring it in a large representative population of normal, healthy individuals, thus obtaining a normal distribution; the central 95% of this normal distribution would then be the "normal range."

Although manufacturers of commercial tests may attempt to establish a reference range by testing thousands, or even tens of thousands of individuals, the practical facts are as follows:

- There is nothing inherently pathologic about the 5% of the population outside this "normal range"; typically, there are some healthy people who have "abnormally" high or low values. Indeed, in some cases an abnormal value—such as a low serum cholesterol value or a high IQ—may be a positive sign rather than a negative one.

- Many biologic variables turn out to be skewed rather than normally distributed in the population.

- The population that is tested to establish the normal range is not usually unambiguously free of disease, because it is difficult to find a large sample of "normal" people who are healthy in every way.

- If this strictly statistical definition of normality and abnormality were adhered to, all diseases would have the same prevalence rate of 5%.

In practice, the normal range and the corresponding reference values presented in a given laboratory's manual often represent a compromise between the statistically derived values and clinical judgment, and may be altered from time to time as the laboratory gains experience with a given test. The values must always be interpreted in the light of other factors that may influence the data obtained about a given patient, such as the patient's age, weight, gender, diet, and the time of day when the specimen was drawn or the measurement made.

SENSITIVITY AND SPECIFICITY

Sensitivity and specificity are both measures of a test's validity—its ability to correctly detect people with or without the disease in question. They are best understood by referring to Table 7–1, which shows the four logical possibilities in diagnostic testing:

TP: A positive test result is obtained in the case of a person who has the disease; this is a "true-positive" finding.

Table 7-1

		DISEASE	
		Present	**Absent**
TEST RESULT	**Positive**	True positive (TP)	False positive (type II error) (FP)
	Negative	False negative (type I error) (FN)	True negative (TN)

FP: A positive test result is obtained in the case of a person who does not have the disease; this finding is therefore a "false-positive" one, which is a type II error.

FN: A negative test result is obtained in the case of a person who does have the disease; this is a "false-negative" result, which constitutes a type I error.

TN: A negative test result is obtained in the case of a person who does not have the disease; this is a "true-negative" result.

Sensitivity

The sensitivity of a test is its ability to detect people who *do* have the disease. It is the percentage of the people with a disease that is correctly detected or classified:

$$\text{Sensitivity} = \frac{\text{number testing positive who have the disease } (TP)}{\text{total number tested who have the disease } (TP + FN)} \times 100$$

Thus, a test that is always positive for individuals with a given disease, identifying *every* person with that disease, has a sensitivity of 100%. Therefore, a test that is insensitive leads to missed diagnoses (false-negative results), whereas a sensitive test produces few false-negative results.

A sensitive test is obviously required in situations in which the consequences of a false-negative result are serious, such as with a serious condition that is treatable or transmissible. Thus, high sensitivity is required of tests used to screen donated blood for human immunodeficiency virus (HIV), for cytologic screening tests (Pap smears) for cervical cancer, and for mammograms.

 Very sensitive tests are therefore used for *screening or ruling out* disease; if the result of a highly sensitive test is negative, it allows the disease to be ruled out with confidence. A mnemonic for this is the word "Snout"—reminding one that a **SeN**sitive test with a **N**egative result rules **OUT** the disease.

Specificity

The specificity of a test is its ability to detect people who **do not** have the disease. It is the percentage of the disease-free people who are correctly classified or detected:

$$\text{Specificity} = \frac{\text{number testing negative who do not have the disease } (TN)}{\text{total number tested who do not have the disease } (FP + TN)} \times 100$$

Thus, a test that is always negative for healthy individuals, identifying *every* nondiseased person, has a specificity of 100%. A test that is low in specificity therefore leads to many false-positive diagnoses, whereas a test that is highly specific produces few false-positive results.

High specificity is required in situations in which the consequences of a false-positive diagnosis are serious. Such situations include those in which the diagnosis may lead to the initiation of dangerous, painful, or expensive treatments (as in the case of cancer chemotherapy); in which a diagnosis may be unduly alarming (HIV, cancer); in which a diagnosis may cause a person to make irreversible decisions (Alzheimer's disease); or in which a diagnosis may result in a person being stigmatized (schizophrenia, HIV, tuberculosis).

 Very specific tests are therefore appropriate for *confirming* or *ruling in* the existence of a disease. If the result of a highly specific test is positive, the disease is almost certainly present. A mnemonic for this is the word "Spin"—reminding one that a **SP**ecific test with a **P**ositive result rules **IN** the disease.

In clinical practice, sensitivity and specificity are inversely related: an increase in one causes a decrease in the other. This is because groups of patients with the disease and groups who are disease-free lie on a continuum, overlapping each other, rather than forming two totally discrete groups. The tester therefore has to select a "cutoff point" to make a diagnostic decision.

For example, the fasting glucose levels of the populations of people who have diabetes and people who do not have diabetes form two overlapping distributions resembling those shown in Figure 7–1.

It is apparent that when a test of the fasting glucose level is used to diagnose diabetes, the choice of cutoff point will determine the test's sensitivity and specificity.

The current generally accepted cutoff point for the diagnosis of diabetes is a fasting glucose level of 126 mg/ml, as shown. This is close to being 100% sensitive—there are a few false-negatives (people with diabetes incorrectly classified as nondiabetic), but not many. There are, however, a substantial number of false positives, so the test is not 100% specific.

If the cutoff point were lowered to 100 mg/100 ml, the test would be 100% sensitive, correctly identifying *every* person with diabetes. Nevertheless, it would have a very low specificity, and the number of false-positive results would be unacceptably high—many persons who do not have diabetes would be incorrectly diagnosed with the disease. As this suggests, highly sensitive tests are likely to have low specificity. Although they correctly classify the vast majority of people with a certain disease (making few false-negative or type I errors), they tend to classify many healthy people incorrectly (making a large number of false-positive or type II errors).

As the cutoff point is increased, it is clear that the test's sensitivity would gradually decrease and its specificity would increase, until the cutoff point reached 150 mg/100 ml, at which point it would be 100% specific. At this level it would correctly identify all persons who do not have diabetes, but it would be highly insensitive, incorrectly diagnosing many persons with diabetes as being free of the disease. Highly specific tests are therefore likely to be associated with a high number of false-negative (type I) errors.

It is clear from Figure 7–1 that a test can only be 100% sensitive *and* 100% specific if there is no overlap between the population that is normal and the population that has the disease. For example, if nobody with diabetes had a fasting glucose level below 130 mg/100 ml, and nobody without diabetes had a level above 120 mg/100 ml, there would be no problem of a tradeoff between sensi-

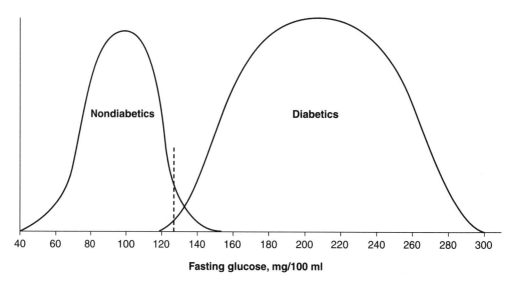

Figure 7-1

tivity and specificity—a cutoff point of 126 mg/100 ml would be perfect. This kind of situation does not occur commonly, and when it does, the disease may be so obvious that no diagnostic testing is required.

 Although there are tests of relatively high sensitivity and specificity for some diseases, it is often best to use a combination of tests when screening for or diagnosing a particular disease. A highly sensitive (and usually relatively cheap) test should be used first, almost guaranteeing the detection of all cases of the disease (albeit at the expense of including a number of false-positive results). This should be followed by a more specific (and usually more expensive) test to eliminate the false-positive results. This is the usual sequence of testing for HIV, hepatitis B, and many other common but serious diseases.

PREDICTIVE VALUES

When the sensitivity of a test is known, it is possible to answer the question, "Given that a patient has the disease, what is the ability of the test to discover this?" When the specificity of a test is known, it is possible to answer the question, "Given that a patient is free of the disease, what is the ability of the test to discover this?"

These are both the kinds of questions that an epidemiologist might ask when screening for a disease. The epidemiologist wants to know, for example, how good a test is at detecting the presence or absence of HIV infection, or what percentage of people with HIV infection will be detected with the test. However, these are not the kinds of questions that the practicing physician or the patient wants answered; when faced with a test result, they want to know how likely it is that the disease really is present or absent. This is a different question altogether, and answering it requires knowledge of the **predictive values** of the test.

Positive predictive value

 The **positive predictive value** (**PPV**) of a test is the proportion of positive results that are true positives, i.e., the likelihood that a person with a positive test result actually has the disease:

$$\text{PPV} = \frac{\text{number who test positive and have the disease } (TP)}{\text{total number who test positive } (TP + FP)}$$

Knowing a test's PPV allows one to answer the question, "Given that the patient's test result is positive, how likely is it that he or she really has the disease?" This is the kind of information that a patient who tests positive (for HIV, for example) wants to know.

Negative predictive value

 The **negative predictive value** (**NPV**) of a test is the proportion of negative results that are true negatives, i.e., the likelihood that a person with a negative result truly does not have the disease:

$$\text{NPV} = \frac{\text{number who test negative and do not have the disease } (TN)}{\text{total number who test negative } (FN + TN)}$$

Knowing a test's NPV allows one to answer the question, "Given that the test result is negative, how likely is it that the disease really is absent?" Once again, this is the kind of information a patient is concerned about.

Whereas the sensitivity and specificity of a test depend only on the characteristics of the test itself, *predictive values vary according to the prevalence (or underlying probability) of the disease*. Thus, predictive values cannot be determined without prior knowledge of the prevalence of the disease—they are not qualities of the test *per se*, but are a function of the test's characteristics and of the setting in which it is being used.

The higher the prevalence of a disease in the population, the higher the PPV and the lower the NPV of a test for it. If a disease is rare, even a very specific test may have a low PPV because it produces a large number of false-positive results. This is an important consideration because many new tests are first used in hospital populations, in which a given disease may be quite common. Hence, a test may produce only a few false-positive results at first but when it is used in the general population (in which the disease may be quite rare), it may produce an unacceptably high proportion of false-positive results.

An example makes the relationship between predictive values and prevalence clearer.

Table 7–2 shows the results of a community-wide HIV screening program, using a test that is 90% sensitive and 99% specific. The community has a population of 10,000, of whom 10 are HIV-positive—so the prevalence of HIV infection is 10 in 10,000, or 0.1%.

Because the test is 90% sensitive, 9 of 10 people with HIV are detected, leaving 1 false-negative result. Because the test is 99% specific, 99% of the uninfected population, or 9890 people, are correctly identified as being free of the virus, leaving 100 false-positive results. What are the predictive values of the test?

- The PPV of the test is $TP/(TP + FP)$, or $9/(9 + 100)$, which is approximately equal to 0.08. This means that there is only an 8% chance that a person with a positive test result actually has the virus.

- The NPV is $TN/(FN + TN)$, or $9890/(1 + 9890) = 0.9999$, meaning that a person with a negative test can be virtually 100% sure that he or she does not have the virus.

If there were an equally sensitive (90%) and specific (99%) test for diabetes, and 1000 people in this population had diabetes, the prevalence would be 1000 per 10,000, or 10%. The results of a screening program for diabetes in the community would be as shown in Table 7–3.

Table 7-2

		HIV INFECTION	
		Present	**Absent**
TEST	**Positive**	9 (*TP*)	100 (*FP*)
RESULT	**Negative**	1 (*FN*)	9890 (*TN*)

Table 7-3

		DIABETES	
		Present	**Absent**
Positive		900 (*TP*)	90 (*FP*)
Negative		100 (*FN*)	8910 (*TN*)

(Row labels on left: T E S T R E S U L T)

Because the test is 90% sensitive, 900 of the 1000 people with diabetes are detected. Because the test is 99% specific, 99% of the 9000 people who do not have diabetes, or 8910 people, will be classified correctly, leaving 90 false-positive results. What are the predictive values of this test, which has exactly the same sensitivity and specificity as the HIV test?

- The PPV of this test is $TP/(TP + FP)$, or 900/990, which is approximately equal to 0.91, meaning that there is a 91% chance that a person with a positive test result actually has diabetes.

- The NPV of the test is $TN/(FN + TN)$, or 8910 + 9010, or approximately 0.99, meaning that there is a 99% chance that a person with a negative test result actually does not have diabetes.

The enormous difference between the PPVs of the tests for diabetes (91%) and HIV (8%) is entirely due to the different prevalences of the two diseases, as the two tests are identical in terms of their sensitivity and specificity. As the prevalence of the disease increases, PPV *increases* and NPV *decreases*.

Because the PPV increases as the prevalence of the disease increases, one way of improving a test's PPV, and hence avoiding a large number of false-positive results, is to restrict its use to high-risk members of the population. For example, if it were decided to use the HIV test only on the 10% of the population who are at the highest risk for HIV, the results might be as shown in Table 7–4.

Referring to the previous example of the HIV screening program, it is now assumed that all 10 HIV infections occurred among members of the high-risk group. Because the test is 90% sensitive, 9 of 10 people with HIV are correctly identified, as before. Because the test is 99% specific, 99% of the 990 uninfected people, or 980 people, are correctly identified, leaving 10 false-positive results. What are the predictive values now?

- The PPV of the test, $TP/(TP + FP)$, is now 9/19, or 0.47 (47%), which is a vast improvement on the previous figure of 8%.

- The NPV of the test, $TN/(TN + FN)$, is 980/981, or approximately 0.99, so it is essentially unchanged.
  Note how the PPV of the test has been enormously improved by limiting its use to high-risk members of the population.

Table 7-4

| | | HIV INFECTION | |
		Present	Absent
T E S T	**Positive**	9 (TP)	10 (FP)
R E S U L T	**Negative**	1 (FN)	980 (TN)

EXERCISES

Select the single, best answer to the following questions.

1. A physician uses an HIV test that, in his population, has a known sensitivity of 99.9%, specificity of 96.9%, positive predictive value of 93.2%, and negative predictive value of 99.7%. Which of these characteristics best permits him to reassure a patient who is worried that the negative HIV test result he has just received may in fact be an error?

a. The sensitivity of the test
b. The specificity of the test
c. The positive predictive value of the test
d. The negative predictive value of the test

2. A test for hepatitis C is performed for 200 patients with biopsy-proven disease and 200 patients known to be free of the disease. The test shows positive results on 180 of the patients with the disease, and negative results on 150 of the patients without the disease. Among those tested, this test therefore

a. has a positive predictive value of 90%.
b. has a negative predictive value of 75%.
c. has a sensitivity of 90%.
d. has a specificity of 82.5%.
e. The information given is insufficient.

3. Due to an effective prevention program, the prevalence of an infectious disease in a community has been reduced by 90%. A physician continues to use the same diagnostic test for the disease that she has always used. How have the test's characteristics changed?

a. Its sensitivity has increased.
b. Its specificity has decreased.

c. Its positive predictive value has increased.
d. Its negative predictive value has increased.
e. The test's characteristics have not changed.

Questions 4 and 5

Select the single, best answer to the questions referring to the following figure.

4. Figure 7–2 shows the distributions of patients who are disease-free and patients who have a certain disease according to their scores on a new quantitative diagnostic test. If the disease in question is fatal if it is not treated, but the treatment is safe and inexpensive, which of the labeled points on the graph represents the best diagnostic cutoff point?

a. A
b. B
c. C
d. D
e. E

5. If the disease in Question 4 universally follows a course of gradual deterioration with eventual death after a period of years, and cannot be treated effectively, which of the labeled points on the graph represents the best diagnostic cutoff point?

a. A
b. B
c. C
d. D
e. E

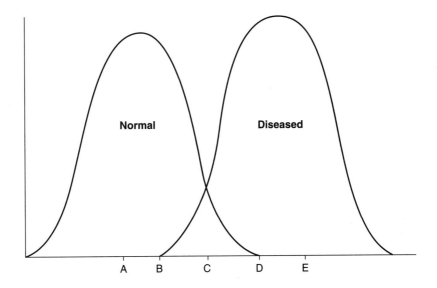

Figure 7-2

Question 6

Select the single, best answer to the following question.

6. A blood transfusion service wishes to screen for an incurable blood-borne disease with a high attack rate. Although its primary responsibility is to the patients who are recipients of its blood, the service is also required to inform blood donors if they are infected with this disease. If there is no test for the disease that is both highly sensitive and highly specific, how should the service test donated blood?

a. With a very sensitive test only
b. With a very specific test only
c. With a very sensitive test initially before blood is sent out to be transfused, and then with a very specific test before informing the donor
d. With a very specific test initially before blood is sent out to be transfused, and then with a very sensitive test before informing the donor

8

Ultra-High-Yield Review

Most USMLE Step 1 candidates probably spend no more than 3 to 5 hours reviewing biostatistics. In this short time, the candidate should be able to memorize the ultra-high-yield items in this checklist. Together with a background understanding from the previous chapters in this book, these items should equip the candidate to pick up a good number of points in a subject area that is neglected by many students and medical schools, which should mean that biostatistics in itself will be relatively a high-yield subject on the examination for the candidate. After this list and the referenced material in this book have been reviewed, a self-test can be administered by using the USMLE-style exercise questions at the end of each chapter.

The USMLE Step 1 candidate should:

- ☐   be able to use the addition and multiplication rules of probability (page 3).
- ☐   be able to find and use the three measures of central tendency (page 11).
    - ☐   mean.
    - ☐   mode.
    - ☐   median.
- ☐   understand the standard deviation (page 13).
- ☐   know and be able to use the proportions of the normal distribution which are within or beyond 1, 2, or 3 standard deviations from the mean (page 13).
- ☐   understand and be able to use z-scores (page 15).
- ☐   understand confidence limits and be able to find 95% confidence limits (page 25).
- ☐   understand precision and accuracy (the dartboard analogy) (page 26).
- ☐   understand how sample size relates to precision (page 26).
- ☐   know exactly how to increase precision and reduce the width of the confidence interval (page 26).
- ☐   know how to be 95% confident about the true mean of a population (page 26).
- ☐   know the meaning and limitations of p values and statistical significance (page 37).
- ☐   know the meaning of type I and type II errors in hypothesis testing and in diagnostic testing (page 37).

☐   know how to avoid type I and type II errors in hypothesis testing (page 37).

☐   know the meaning of a test's power, how to increase it, and the dangers of a lack of power (the radar screen analogy) (pages 37–38).

☐   know the meaning of main and interaction effects in ANOVA (the beards and lipstick analogy) (page 44).

☐   know the use of chi-square (page 46).

☐   know the meaning and use of correlation coefficients and r values (page 50).

☐   be able to avoid the temptation to infer causation from correlation (page 52).

☐   be able to interpret scattergrams of bivariate distributions (page 51).

☐   calculate and know the meaning of the coefficient of determination (r^2) (page 52).

☐   know what regression techniques do (pages 52–53).

☐   memorize Table 4–1 to be able to choose the appropriate basic test for a given research question (page 54).

☐   know the purposes of the features of clinical trials: (pages 59–60)

    ☐   control groups.

    ☐   blinding.

    ☐   randomization or matching.

☐   know the advantages, disadvantages, and typical uses of:

    ☐   cohort studies (the Framingham study and chimney sweeps example) (pages 62–63).

    ☐   case-control studies (DES and vaginal carcinoma study) (page 63).

    ☐   case series studies (page 64).

    ☐   prevalence surveys (page 64).

☐   be able to choose the appropriate type of research study for a given question (pages 62–64).

☐   know the meanings of and be able to find: (pages 68–69)

    ☐   incidence.

    ☐   prevalence.

    ☐   morbidity.

    ☐   mortality.

    ☐   and the relationships between them (the epidemiologist's bathtub) (page 70).

☐   know the meaning of case-fatality and attack rates (page 70).

☐   know the meanings of and be able to find: (pages 72–73)

    ☐   absolute risk and absolute risk reduction.

☐   relative risk and relative risk reduction.

☐   number needed to treat.

☐   know the meaning of validity (including internal and external validity) and reliability (page 78–79).

☐   know the meanings of and be able to find:

☐   sensitivity (page 81).

☐   specificity (page 81).

☐   positive predictive value (page 83).

☐   negative predictive value (page 83).

☐   know how changing a test's cutoff point will affect its sensitivity and specificity (page 82).

☐   know what kind of test to use to rule in or rule out a disease (mnemonics "Snout" and "Spin") (page 81).

Appendix 1: Statistical Symbols

Symbols are listed in order of their appearance in the text.

X — A single element

N — Number of elements in a population

n — Number of elements in a sample

p — The probability of an event occurring. In reports of statistical significance, p is the probability that the result could have been obtained by chance—i.e., the probability that a type I error is being made

q — The probability of an event not occurring; equal to $(1 - p)$

f — Frequency

C — Centile (or percentile) rank; or confidence level

Mo — Mode

Mdn — Median

μ — Population mean

$\overline{X}$ — Sample mean

Σ — The sum of

χ — Deviation score

σ^2 — Population variance

S^2 — Sample variance

σ — Population standard deviation (SD)

S — Sample standard deviation (SD)

z — The number of standard deviations by which a single element in a normally distributed population lies from the population mean; or the number of standard errors by which a random sample mean lies from the population mean

$\mu_{\overline{x}}$ — The mean of the random sampling distribution of means

$\sigma_{\overline{x}}$ — Standard error or standard error of the mean (standard deviation of the random sampling distribution of means) [SEM or SE]

$s_{\overline{x}}$ — Estimated standard error (estimated standard error of the mean)

t — The number of estimated standard errors by which a random sample mean lies from the population mean

df — Degrees of freedom

α — The criterion level at which the null hypothesis will be accepted or rejected; the probability of making a type I error

β — Probability of making a type II error

F — A ratio of variances

χ^2 — Chi-square; a test of proportions

r — Correlation coefficient

ρ — Rho; Spearman rank order correlation coefficient

r^2 — Coefficient of determination

b — Regression coefficient; the slope of the regression line

Appendix 2: Exercise Answers

CHAPTER 1

1. **d**—Bias occurs when a result consistently errs in a particular direction. If the sample is drawn from smokers who come to the physician's office, and these patients are likely to smoke more than those who do not come to the physician's office, then the result will consistently tend to overestimate the number of cigarettes smoked by all the smokers in the practice. Systematic samples can be as representative as simple random samples.

2. **d**—The multiplication rule of probability tells us that the probability of two or more independent events all occurring is equal to the product of their individual probabilities. The probability of one patient being a smoker is 20% (0.2), and the probability of the next patient being a smoker is also 0.2; so the probability of two smokers appearing in succession is 0.2×0.2, or 0.04.

3. **a**—The addition rule of probability tells us that the probability of any one of several particular events occurring is equal to the sum of their individual probabilities. The probability of a patient being a smoker is 20% (0.2), and the probability of a patient being a woman is 0.5; so the probability of the next patient being a smoker or a woman is $0.2 + 0.5 = 0.7$.

4. **d**—The number of cigarettes smoked constitutes a ratio scale—there is an absolute zero, and meaningful ratios do exist. It is discrete data, not continuous—as the physician is counting the whole number of cigarettes smoked.

5. **a**—The frequency distribution has been stated to be a normal distribution, and in any normal distribution the three measures of central tendency (mean, mode, and median) will all be coincident (as shown in Fig. 1–9).

6. **d**—The deviation score (x) corresponding to smoking 24 cigarettes is 8, as 24 minus the mean (16) is 8.

7. **c**—The physician is finding the mean of the squares of the deviation scores, which is the definition of variance.

8. **d**—Standard deviation is the square root of the variance, and 4 is the square root of 16.

9. **b**—The z-score of an element is the number of standard deviations by which the element lies above (positive z-scores) or below (negative z-scores) the mean. In this case, the mean is 16, and the standard deviation is 4, so an element with a value of 24 or 2 standard deviations lies above the mean.

10. **a**—Twenty-four cigarettes corresponds to a z-score of $+2$, as shown in Question 9. For all normal distributions, 2.5% of the distribution lies above a z-score of $+2$, so 2.5% of smokers in this population smoke more than 24 cigarettes per day, as shown in Figure 1-1.

11. **d**—Twenty cigarettes a day corresponds to a z-score of $+1$ (as 20 lies 1 standard deviation above the mean, 16); as 68% of the distribution lies between z-scores of $+1$ and -1, 32%

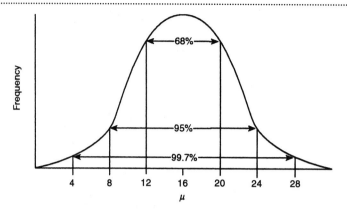

Figure A-1

lies in the "tails" of the distribution, beyond these points. Normal distributions are symmetrical by definition, so 16% of the distribution must lie above $z = +1$.

12. **d**—Twelve cigarettes a day corresponds to a z-score of -1 (as 12 lies 1 standard deviation below the mean, 16). As seen in the answer to Question 11, 16% of the distribution lies below this score. This means that the probability of the next (presumably random) smoker smoking less than 12 cigarettes per day is also 16%, or .16.

13. **c**—Table 1–3 shows that the z-score that divides the top 5% of the distribution from the remaining 95% is approximately $+1.65$. The score (or number of cigarettes) corresponding to this z-score is therefore the mean, (16) plus 1.65 standard deviations (4), or $16 + 6.6 = 22.6$, or approximately 23.

CHAPTER 2

1. **e**—The research problem clearly involves the use of inferential statistics. It would be impractical to weigh every adult male New Yorker (b), and therefore only a sample of New Yorkers should be weighed. The central limit theorem tells us that as long as the sample is random (d or e), it does not matter that the underlying population may not be normally distributed; so (a) is not necessary. A larger sample (e) is clearly preferable to a smaller one (d).

2. **a**—Random samples that are drawn from the population of interest will be accurate (unbiased); hence a and b are likely to be accurate. Samples that are drawn from a nonrandom subset of the population, such as joggers (c and d) will be inaccurate or biased (joggers may be likely to weigh less than other members of the population). Large samples (a) will give precise estimates, whereas small samples (b) will give imprecise estimates.

3. **c**—Estimated standard error is equal to the sample standard deviation (15) divided by the square root of $(n-1)$; with $n = 101$, the estimated standard error is therefore 1.5.

4. **b**—The 95% confidence limits are equal to the mean (72) plus or minus approximately 2 standard errors (2×1.5), or 69 and 75.

5. **b**—The width of the confidence interval is $(75 - 69)$ or 6.

6. **d**—To halve the width of the confidence interval, standard error needs to be halved, and the only way to do this is by quadrupling n.

7. **b**—Halving the width of the confidence interval is the same as doubling precision, as the degree to which the estimate is affected by random variation has halved. Bias has not been reduced, as this is dependent on the truly random quality of the sample.

8. **e**—The new estimate will be more precise (because the standard deviation is less, and hence the estimated standard error and the width of the confidence interval will be reduced), but it is less accurate (because of the biased nature of the sample).

9. **c**— Although the oncologist's predictions were precise, their estimates clearly erred in a consistently pessimistic direction and were therefore biased.

CHAPTER 3

1. **c**—The p value is the probability that the result could be due to chance, rather than due to a real effect; thus, if the drug were ineffective, there is still a .05 chance that this result could have been obtained. The researchers are 95% certain that the drug is effective, and the study is clearly powerful enough to detect an effect, as one was detected. Because the p value is $\leq$ .05, the result is statistically significant.

2. **d**—Once again, the p value is the probability that the result could be due to chance, and it is therefore the probability that the null hypothesis is being rejected incorrectly—the probability of making a type I or false-negative error. As a significant result was obtained, and the null hypothesis rejected, the sample size clearly was adequate.

3. **b**—Chi-square is a test of proportion or nominal scale data (e.g., number or proportion of immunized patients developing zoster versus number or proportion of nonimmunized patients developing zoster). None of the other hypotheses involve tests of proportion or involve nominal scale data.

4. **c**—ANOVA is used when comparisons are being made between multiple group means. Hypotheses involving just two means (a, e) are best tested with a t-test, whereas those involving proportions or frequencies of nominal data (b, d) are best tested with a chi-square test

5. **b**—As the sample drawn is random, the central limit theorem tells us that the sample mean is a member of a normal distribution (the random sampling distribution of means), irrespective of the shape of the underlying population distribution. All the other answers are correct.

6. **d**—Reducing alpha, or making the decision criterion more stringent, allows one to be more confident that any significant results are not due to chance. However, it reduces the likelihood that statistically significant results will be obtained (a), makes a type II error more likely (as it increases the likelihood of accepting the null hypothesis) (b), and makes a type I error less likely (as it decreases the likelihood of rejecting the null hypothesis) (c). The power of the test is reduced by making alpha more stringent (e).

7. **a**—An inability to obtain a statistically significant finding may be due to a sample size that is too small (a lack of power)—not one that is too large, which will increase the likelihood of statistical significance.

CHAPTER 4

1. **b**—The percentage of variance in one variable accounted for by the other is r^2, or $0.8 \times 0.8 = 0.64$. Correlation does not imply causality, so increasing the value of one variable (at-

tending class more) will not necessarily increase the value of the other (grade). A correlation coefficient of 0.8 is considered to be high, and the low p value means it is statistically significant. Although there may be a nonlinear correlation, there clearly is a strong linear one, as the Pearson technique is strictly linear.

2. **e**—Correlation coefficients vary from a minimum -1.00 to a maximum of $+1.00$, indicating perfect negative and positive correlations, respectively. The lecturer is clearly in error.

3. **a**—This constitutes a nominal (or categorical) division of data; the groups are simply named.

4. **c**—Chi-square is used to test hypotheses concerning differences between proportions or frequencies in categories.

5. **a**—This problem involves making comparisons of ratio scale data (survival time) across multiple groups, and ANOVA is therefore appropriate.

6. **c**—Regression is used to determine a quantitative relationship which permits the value of one variable to be used to predict the value of another.

7. **b**—The correlation is strong (0.7), positive, and statistically significant. Correlation in itself does not demonstrate a causal relationship, so it provides no evidence that work satisfaction or enjoying one's work will cause one to live longer. Nor does it provide any indication as to what percentage of people who enjoy their work have above-average life expectancy. The proportion of variability in life expectancy that can be mathematically accounted for by work satisfaction is $r^2 = 0.49$ or 49%.

8. **c**—A correlation coefficient alone does not demonstrate causality; there could be other reasons why there is a relationship between drug dosage and blood pressure. The low p value shows that the finding is unlikely to be due to chance (a); a correlation coefficient of -0.3 is a weak negative one (b); drug dosage accounts for $r^2 = 0.09$ or 9% of the variation in blood pressures (d); and regression techniques would allow a quantitative prediction to be made (e).

9. **b**—Overall, the drugs have no effect nor does the gender of the patient; the answer to whether the drugs have any effects at all is "it depends" (on the type of drug and the gender of the patient), showing that there is an interaction between the drug and the gender of the patient. Although there are no main effects (c, d, and e), it is incorrect to say that there are no effects at all (a).

CHAPTER 5

1. **d**—Cohort studies start with a group of people who do not have the disease of interest, and follow them over time to see which of them subsequently develop the disease. All the other research methods generally include at least some patients who have the disease of interest; the only exception might be a clinical trial of a treatment intended to prevent the disease.

2. **c**—Control groups help to eliminate alternative explanations for the results of the study. If 75% of patients given a certain treatment recover from an illness, it could be argued that these patients would have recovered anyway (spontaneous remission). However, if only 20% of a comparable control group recovered, this alternative explanation is not tenable.

3. **a**—The random assignment of patients to experimental and control groups aims to equalize the effects of extraneous variables (such as age and disease severity), so that patients in the two groups are comparable.

4. **b**—Cohort studies are the most powerful form of nonexperimental study and are the best alternative to controlled experiments. They are the only means of determining the absolute

risk of contracting a disease, and their assessment of risk factors is not biased by outcome or recall.

5. **a**—This is a randomly controlled clinical trial, as the patients are randomly allocated to the control and treatment groups. It is double-blind, not single-blind, as neither the patients nor the treating physicians are aware of this allocation.

6. **c**—The biggest failing in this study is that patient gender is a confounding factor, and it will not be possible to know if any difference between the treatment and control groups is due to the treatment or to the gender of the patients. Random allocation of patients to the two groups would have partly or entirely overcome this problem. This study is an experiment, and it does have a dependent variable (reduction in symptoms) and an independent variable (administration of the drug). A double-blind design would also have been advantageous, but its absence is not as serious an error as the problem of confounding and lack of randomization.

7. **e**—This is a case-control study. The 150 children with the disease are cases, and the 300 disease-free children are the controls. Thus, it is a retrospective study, looking at past events. There is no intervention, so it is not a controlled clinical trial.

8. **b**—Case-control studies look back at past events and are therefore retrospective.

9. **b**—Case-control studies are suitable for seeking the cause of very rare diseases, as they study patients who already have the disease.

10. **a**—Cohort studies are expensive, and it may be several or many years before enough members of the cohort develop the disease(s) of interest.

11. **a**—Cohort studies are the only way of establishing the absolute risk of contracting a disease.

12. **e**—Controlled clinical trials typically use random allocation of participants to different groups, such as to treatment and control groups.

13. **b**—Case-control studies are a quick and cheap way of helping to find the cause of the disease even when only a few subjects are available. They present no significant ethical problems because the researcher does not intervene to change a situation, but looks back into the past at events that have already happened.

14. **e**—Controlled clinical trials are the most powerful way of establishing cause-and-effect relationships.

15. **a**—Cohort studies are also known as prospective studies, as they look forward for diseases or events that have not yet occurred.

CHAPTER 6

1. **a**—It will decrease the prevalence of the disease, as prevalence is equal to incidence times the average duration of the disease. The incidence is unchanged because the number of new cases is unchanged.

2. **d**—Twenty of 160 cases resulted in death, so the case-fatality rate is 20/160 or 12.5%, meaning that 12.5% of all cases of pulmonary embolism resulted in death. The rate refers to the proportion of cases resulting in death, not to the number of cases or deaths per annum.

3. **e**—Improving the prevention of a disease will obviously decrease the number of new cases (incidence) of the disease. The "epidemiologist's bathtub" should be recalled: reducing the

flow of water into the bathtub will clearly also result in reduced levels of water (reduced prevalence) if all other factors remain unchanged.

4. **a**—The absolute risk of the disease is the same as its incidence, which in the placebo group is 40 in 1000, or 4%.

5. **c**—The absolute risk of the disease is the same as its incidence, which in the drug group is 10 in 1000, or 1%.

6. **c**—The relative risk of the disease in those who took the drug is 1.0/4.0 or 0.25. This means that patients exposed to the drug had 25% of the risk of cancer of those who took the placebo. The relative risk reduction is therefore $1 - 0.25 = 0.75$ or 75%.

7. **c**—The absolute risk reduction is the difference between the absolute risk or incidence in the control group (4%) and the absolute risk or incidence in the drug group (1%)—so it is 3%. Note the difference between the absolute risk reduction of 3% and the *relative* risk reduction of 75%.

8. **d**—The absolute risk reduction in breast cancer was 3%—in other words, of 100 women treated, 3 fewer would have contracted breast cancer. The number needed to treat to prevent one case is therefore 33.3.

9. **d**—The drug costs $100 per month, or $1200 per annum, or $6000 over the 5 years of the study. As 33.3 patients needed to be treated for 5 years to prevent one case of breast cancer, the cost of preventing one case is $6000 \times 33.3 = \$200,000$.

CHAPTER 7

1. **d**—The negative predictive value is the proportion of negative results that are true negatives. The patient can be told that it is 99.7% certain that he does not have HIV.

2. **c**—This type of question is best answered by constructing a 2×2 table along the lines of Table 7–2. The test is 90% sensitive, because it correctly identifies 180 patients (true positives) out of the total of 200 patients who do have the disease. It is 75% specific, as it correctly identifies 150 (true negatives) out of a total of 200 patients who do not have the disease. Its PPV is the proportion of patients with positive test results who actually have the disease [true positives/(true positives + false positives)] = 180/230 = 78.3%. Its NPV is the proportion of patients with negative test results that truly do not have the disease [true negatives/(false negatives + true negatives)] = 150/170 = 88.2%.

3. **d**—The NPV of the test will increase due to the decreased prevalence of the disease, as there will be fewer false negatives. The PPV will decrease; even a quite sensitive test can produce an unacceptable number of false positives when it is used for a rare disease. Sensitivity and specificity are inherent characteristics of a test which do not change according to the context in which the test is used.

4. **b**—As the disease is fatal if untreated, the consequences of a type I (false-negative) diagnostic error are catastrophic: a patient will be incorrectly diagnosed as not having the disease and will die as a result. The cutoff for diagnosis should therefore be set at a point that guarantees 100% sensitivity, which is point B. In this example, there is no significant penalty for type II (false-positive) diagnostic errors, as treating patients who do not actually have the disease is safe and inexpensive.

5. **d**—The dismal prognosis means that it is essential to avoid making a type II (false-positive) diagnostic error. The cutoff point should therefore be set at a point that guarantees high

specificity, so that no patient without the disease is incorrectly diagnosed with it. As there is no treatment, the consequences of making a type I error, and telling a person with the disease that he or she does not have it, are not severe. Alzheimer's disease is one example of this kind of disease.

6. c—The primary requirement is for a very sensitive test to rule out the disease (Snout) so that the blood can be given safely to a recipient. If this first test result is positive, the blood will not be used, but as a very sensitive but nonspecific test will have a substantial number of false positives, the donor should not be informed that he has the disease until it has been ruled in (Spin) by a second test that is very specific rather than sensitive. This is the typical sequence of testing done for HIV and hepatitis C.

References

Herbst AL, Ulfelder H, Poskanzer DC: Adenocarcinoma of the vagina: Association of maternal stilbestrol therapy with tumor appearance in young women. *N Engl J Med* 284: 878–881, 1971.

Hill OW Jr: Rethinking the "significance" of the rejected null hypothesis. *Am Psychol* 45: 667–668, 1990.

Lipid Research Clinics Program: The Coronary Primary Prevention Trial: Design and implementation. *J Chronic Dis* 32: 609–631, 1979.

Rubin DH, Krasnilkoff PA, Leventhal JM, et al: Effect of passive smoking on birth-weight. *Lancet* ii: 415–417, 1986.

Shepherd J, Cobbe SM, Ford I, et al: Prevention of coronary heart disease with pravastatin in men with hypercholesterolemia. *N Engl J Med* 333: 1301–1307, 1995.

Zito RA, Reid PR: Lidocaine kinetics predicted by indocyanine green clearance. *N Engl J Med* 298: 1160–1163, 1978.

Index

References in *italics* indicate figures; those followed by "t" denote tables